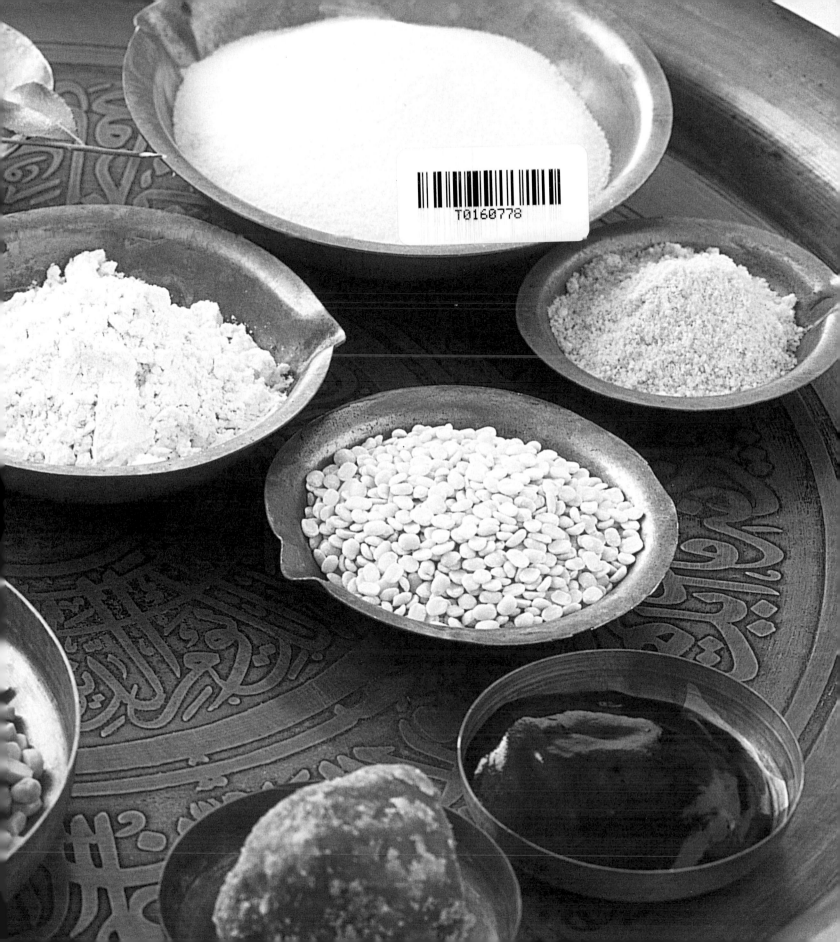

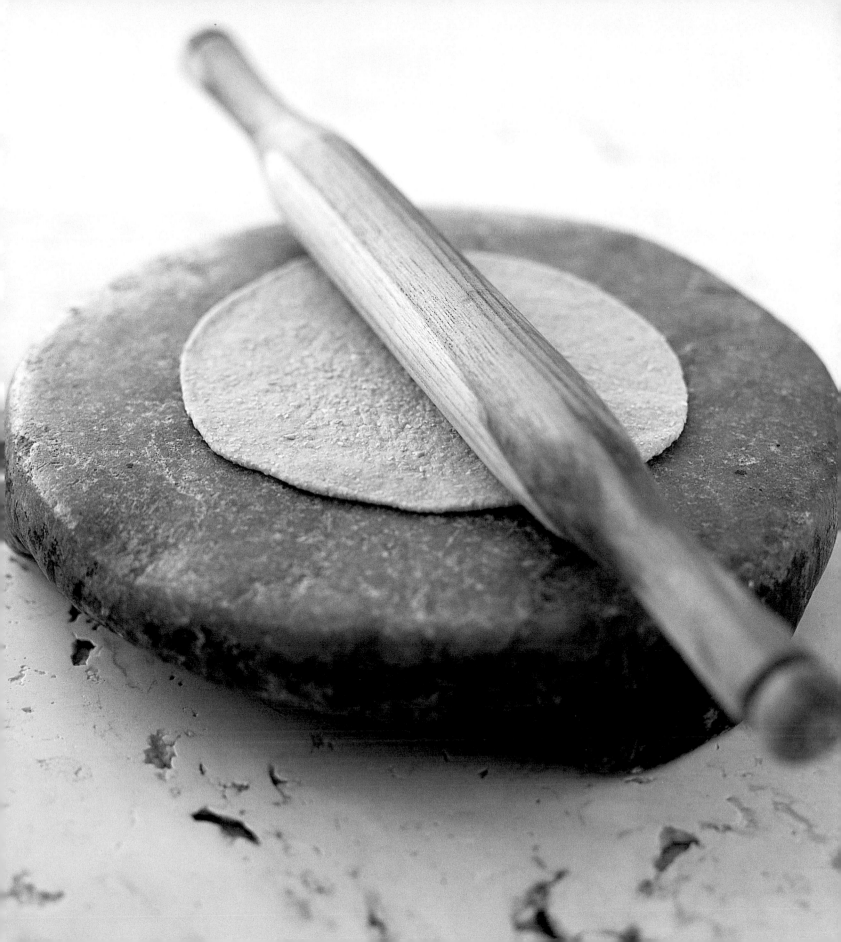

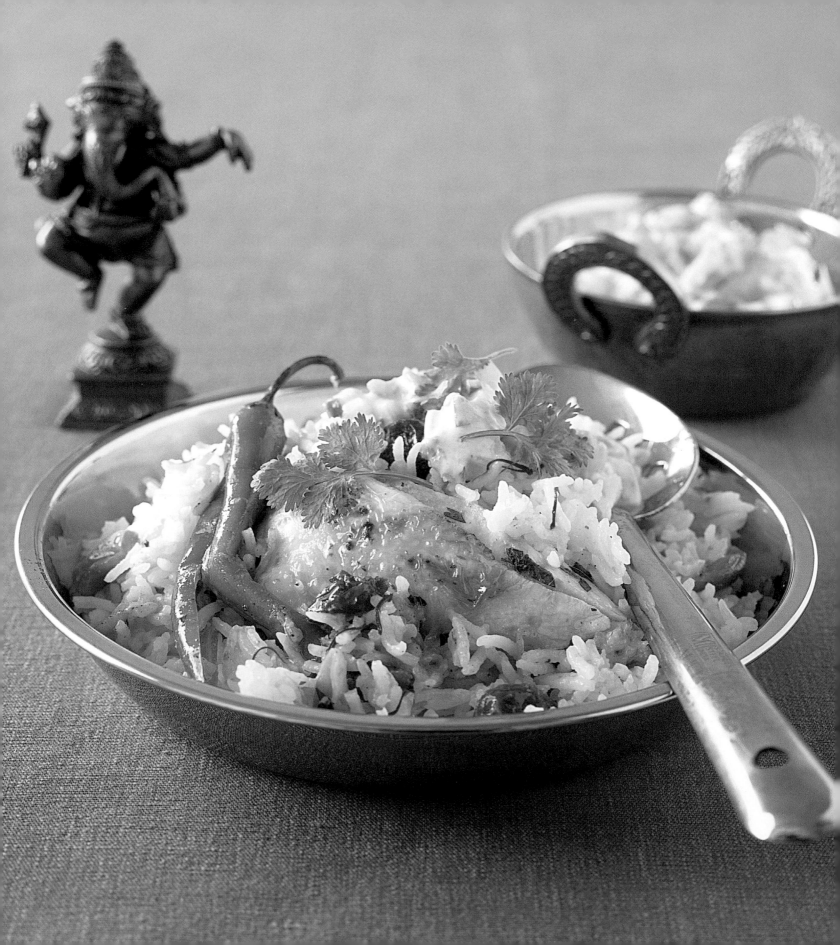

Regional Indian Cooking

Ajoy Joshi and Alison Roberts

PERIPLUS

First published in the United States in 2006 by Periplus Editions (HK) Ltd.,
with editorial offices at 364 Innovation Drive, North Clarendon, VT 05759 and
130 Joo Seng Road, #06-01/03 Singapore 368357

Text, photography and design © 2005 Lansdowne Publishing Pty. Ltd.

ISBN-13 978-0-7946-5025-4
ISBN-10 0-7946-5025-2
Printed in Singapore

DISTRIBUTED BY

North America and Latin America (English Language)
Tuttle Publishing
364 Innovation Drive, North Clarendon, VT 05759-9436
Tel: (802) 773-8930 Fax: (802) 773-6993
Email: info@tuttlepublishing.com
www.tuttlepublishing.com

Japan
Tuttle Publishing
Yaekari Building 3F, 5-4-12 Osaki,
Shinagawa-ku, Tokyo 141-0032
Tel: (03) 5437-0171 Fax: (03) 5437-0755
Email: tuttle-sales@gol.com

Asia Pacific
Berkeley Books (Pte) Ltd
130 Joo Seng Road #06-01/03
Singapore 368357
Tel: (65) 6280-1330 Fax: (65) 6280-6290
Email: inquiries@periplus.com.sg
www.periplus.com

Commissioned by Deborah Nixon
Text: Ajoy Joshi, Alison Roberts and Antonia Beattie
Photographer: Steve Brown
Stylist: Michelle Noerianto
Food preparation: Christine Sheppard and Saskia Hay
Designer: Robyn Latimer
Editor: Sharon Silva
Project Coordination: Bettina Hodgson and Sally Hurworth
Production: Sally Stokes and Eleanor Cant
Photography credits: The Ceramic Shed, Country Floors, Ruby Star Traders

Set in Stone Sans on QuarkXPress

Acknowledgments: Special thanks to Ruby Star Traders, Sydney, Australia, for assistance
with photography

A Special Dedication

I would like to dedicate this book, my second cookbook, to my father who lived and died his own way. He was a scientist in the field of organic chemistry who particularly loved helping guide postgraduate and doctorate students in the completion of their theses in this area.

As I was on my way to Mumbhai en route to Nagpur six days after he died, I had to do my final proofread of this book before it needed to be sent to the publisher for printing and I thought of him – he would have loved to have been able to help.

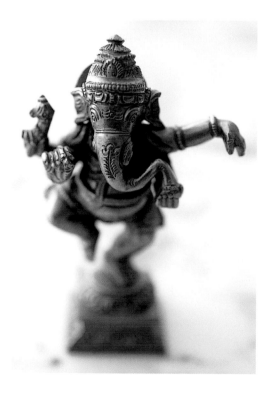

Contents

Introduction

Mangalorean chicken, Punjabi black-eyed beans, cottage cheese dumplings in rose water and saffron syrup, shrimp balchao, and Hyderabadi-style fish stew are just some of the mouthwatering recipes in this cookbook, which is my personal celebration of some of the best regional dishes from the different parts of India. Although there are nearly 28 states in India, five main regions can be discerned – the North, South, East, West and Central regions. Each region contains a number of states and communities. Not surprisingly, each region, as a result of its distinctive geography, agriculture and the communities' lifestyles, offers a unique cuisine.

Although it is impossible to include every dish of each region, the 120 dishes I have chosen as my favorites will give cooks of all levels an excellent insight into the various culinary delights of each region. The regional cooking of India is a fascinating topic that would take several lifetimes to fully appreciate and disseminate. I hope to have yet another lifetime in which to create a third cookbook that honors this type of cooking.

The beauty of Indian regional cooking is that it celebrates the produce and lifestyle of each region – it is the food of the land and the people. The climatic extremes of the North have led to the development of both rich dishes for the winter and simple dishes for the summer. Tandoori and Korma dishes predominate in this region. The South is famous for its hot and spicy foods, in particular the peppery Madras "Kari." The East, which is close to the Chinese border, specializes in chili curries and dishes with

tamarind and mustard oil. The West boasts a host of coconut and seafood dishes while the Central region of India, which is the place to which I belong, has taken the best of all of the other four regions and has created a subtle cuisine, which is rich, yet light on the stomach.

At a deeper level, Indian cooking also echoes a number of ancient beliefs concerning the interrelationship between food and the health of the body. Many centuries ago, a sophisticated system of health and life was developed, which is still practiced today, called Ayurveda. Ayurvedic medicine is a holistic form of healing and its practitioners believe, among other things, that different foods have healing qualities for certain types of people.

Food can be seen as a double-edged sword in Ayurvedic medicine; it can cause disease as well as prevent it. Eaten in the right quantities and in the right form, different dishes can be extremely good for the body. The food is broken down by the gastric juices of the body and its nutrients are easily absorbed. However, if the balance is disturbed and the food cannot be digested easily, the same dishes can cause an imbalance, which could lead to "tensions."

In Ayurvedic medicine, the undigested food particles that cause these tensions can be rectified using a therapy that rebalances the body through an understanding of the interactions between the five elements of nature – Fire (*Agni*), Earth (*Bhoomi*), Air (*Vayu*), Water (*Jal*), and Space or Ether (*Akash*). Ayurvedic practitioners believe that the combination and balance between these five elements determine the characteristics of our body, health and personalities and affect how our organs work.

It is believed that each person is predominantly one of three body types (*prakruti*). These body types are called kapha, pitta and vata. Each body type is governed by the interaction of two elements. A kapha type of person, who is generally a large-boned person with brown eyes and hair, is a combination of Earth and Water. A pitta body type, who is usually fair or red-haired and of medium build, is a combination of Fire and Water. A vata type of person, who is usually slim and wiry with dark hair, is a combination of Space or Ether and Air. It is believed that each body type has certain preferences for foods. A dish that will be easy for a vata type to digest would not be suitable for a kapha type person. This is a fascinating topic and I will say more about it in my special Elements section before the start of the recipes.

Knowledge of these elements is a very powerful healing tool and is interrelated with an understanding of many other aspects of life, such as colors and directions of the compass. These interrelationships between the elements and other areas of life also occur in other ancient civilizations, such as that of China. In my restaurant I have developed a series of five rooms, each honoring an element. Further I have assigned an element for each region: the North region is Earth, the South is Fire, the East is Air, the West is Water, and the Central region is Space or Ether. I decorated each room with the appropriate colors and pictures from the region, and in each room I included a menu featuring dishes from that specific region.

The dishes I have chosen for this book are extremely straightforward. I follow a very simple philosophy that there must be a balance between salt (*uppu* or *namak*), a souring agent (*puli* or *khatas*) and chili (*karam* or *mirchi*). Once you add a sense of relaxation or leisure (*fursat*) and some love (*mohabbat*), you will find that you have prepared the perfect dish!

Cooking Indian food, like any other great cuisine, is a fabulous celebration of life. The recipes in this book are a selection of popular or notable dishes, presented in a format that makes them easy to prepare. I have included a section on simple cooking techniques and how to prepare our famous garam marsala, as well as the basic spice mixtures for each of the five regions. I hope you enjoy the journey of cooking each dish as much as the pleasure of eating it. Finally, as any self-respecting Indian would say at the conclusion of a good meal:

"Anha datha Sukhi Bhava"
May the provider of this food be happy and content!

Ajoy Joshi

About Regional Cooking

I have always had a love of good food, even as a young boy. I first became involved in the hospitality industry in India in the late 70s, starting out in a catering school in Madras and then working with the Taj Group, the largest chain of hotels in India. I learnt my calling as a chef there, starting as an apprentice cook at Fisherman's Cove Hotel, and it was through the Taj Group that I eventually met my future wife, who was also working as a chef.

While working with the Taj Group in the banquet kitchen, I became aware that there was still quite a limited range of Indian dishes available on a commercial level – there had to be more! I was particularly inspired by the Usha restaurant in Mangalore, which was one of the first restaurants to provide Indian home-style cooking, focusing on the food of that region of India.

In 1988, I achieved one of my dreams as I was appointed executive chef of the Gateway Hotel in Bangalore. The Taj Group then allowed me the chance to travel to various regions, such as Malabar, and to eventually start the Karavalli restaurant in Bangalore.

I moved to Australia in 1988 and started a chain of five Indian restaurants in Brisbane called the Scherhazade. After returning to India to marry Meera, I came back with her to Australia and in 1992 started a restaurant in Sydney called The Malabar, in honor of one of the areas where I had worked in India. The restaurant was very successful, but we grew restless and eventually sold the business, afterwards taking some time to travel the world.

In 1997, my wife and I felt that we would like to return to the restaurant industry and decided to open an Indian restaurant in Sydney that focused on regional Indian cooking. We were very keen that the restaurant had some form of connection between the regions of India and that Sydney was highlighted. This is why we named the restaurant Nilgiri's, which is an Indian term that translates as the "Blue Mountains," a mountain range that is just two hours west of Sydney. It is also the name of a mountain range in the southwest of India.

Achieving yet another dream, my first cookery book was launched at Nilgiri's on 3 March 2003. It was inevitable that a second book would be written! However, after almost six years at Crows Nest, Sydney, we decided to relocate Nilgiri's to new premises in St Leonards, Sydney. The relocation was a dream project for us.

Although the first month on the new premises boded well, things started falling apart and we focused on redeveloping our restaurant. We realized that we needed to have an open plan kitchen – something that Nilgiri's at Crows Nest had made its own for nearly six years. Now that this has been implemented and business has improved dramatically, I have been able to focus on creating a new cookbook.

My writing partner on the first book, Jan Purser, was a great encouragement. However, when she was unable to continue with the project due to her relocation to Perth, I was fortunate to meet Alison Roberts, who was extremely patient, calm, focused and committed. She has been a great person to work with and the book has really come into existence due to her dedication. I would also like to thank Lansdowne for being more than willing to be the publisher of this book.

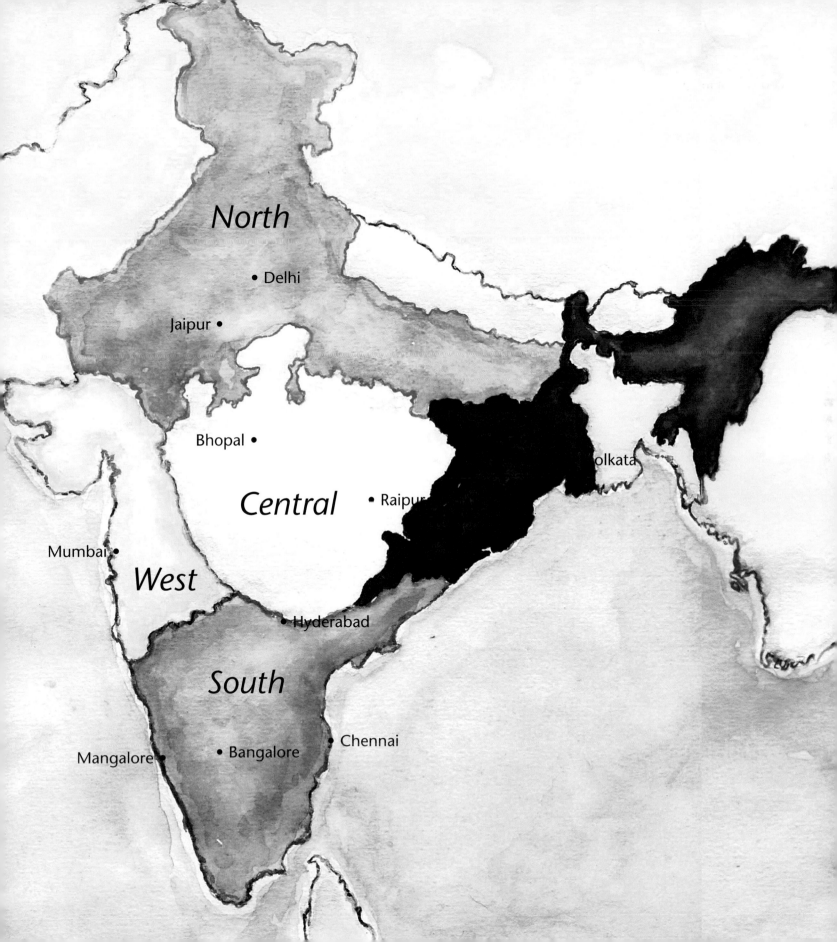

The Elements
and How They Affect Your Dining Pleasure

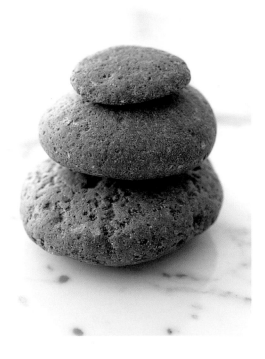

Introduction
The healing qualities of Indian cuisine

Indian cooking has evolved over many centuries and has incorporated a number of influences from other nations. It also reflects a number of important concepts from one of the oldest forms of holistic healing known in the world. The ancient science of life, which is known as Ayurveda, is still widely practised today. Ayurvedic practitioners believe that the proper consumption of the right amount and the correct type of food helps to maintain a person's health. However, eating the wrong quantity, quality and type of food may cause disease. Most of the diseases we know are either directly or indirectly caused by the food we eat.

One of the most important functions of the human body is believed to be the digestion. If our food is not digested well, we find that toxins build up in the body and get in the way of the body functioning properly, causing disease and other complications. So, at the bottom line, it is food that decides the functioning of the human body. If we do not digest our food properly, Ayurvedic practitioners often suggest an array of therapies and spices to help balance the body's chemistry so that there is enough fire (or *agni*) in the body to digest the food you eat.

Spices and certain tastes are introduced in the diet to help a person digest their food. In Ayurvedic medicine, six kinds of tastes are identified – sweet, sour, salty, pungent, bitter and astringent. Each kind of taste is associated with two of five elements.

In Ayurveda, five elements are believed to make up everything in the universe. These elements are known as Earth, Air, Fire, Water, and Space or Ether. Virtually all things can be described in terms of what elements are believed to be predominant in them, even people. There are three types of constitutions or *prakruti* in Ayurvedic medicine – kapha, pitta and vata types.

Tastes	Corresponding foods and spices
Sweet	Rice, wheat, sugar, milk
Sour	Lemon, vinegar, tamarind, tomato
Salty	Salt
Pungent	Chilies, onion, garlic, mustard seed
Astringent	Lentils, beans, broccoli, cabbage
Bitter	Turmeric, horseradish, endive, spinach

In Ayurvedic beliefs, a person who has a kapha constitution (a balance of Earth and Water) will usually need astringent, pungent or bitter tastes to help rebalance his or her digestion. A vata type person, who is a balance between Space and Air, will need sweet, sour or salty tastes to help with his or her digestion. A person with a pitta constitution (a balance between Fire and Water) will need some sweet, bitter or astringent flavors in their dish to help aid their digestion.

The whole meal does not have to predominantly taste bitter or astringent, it should simply have a bitter or astringent ingredient or two. Most regional Indian dishes include a wider range of tastes that balance with each other than Western culinary food – it is exciting to explore how such flavors can not only taste good but be good for you!

The chart on page 14 lists some characteristics that may help you determine your constitution and what food will best suit it. You may be a combination of body types – for instance, you may have blond hair and a large frame, which might mean that you are a kapha/pitta type. If you are interested in this fascinating area, you might wish to contact an Ayurvedic practitioner for a more in-depth assessment of your constitution and state of health.

We'll go through each element and look at what other therapies can further help you improve your digestion and enhance your enjoyment of your meal.

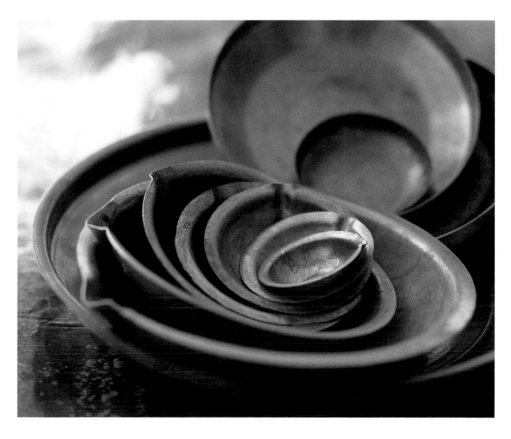

Constitution type	Characteristics of type	Suitable foods
Kapha type	Heavy or large body frame	Basmati rice
	Wide shoulders and hips	Ghee
	Easily tanned skin	Apples, pears, figs
	Medium or dark brown hair	Pumpkin, spinach, broccoli
	Soft brown eyes	Beans
	Heavy sleeper	Chicken, turkey and shrimp
	Compassionate, friendly personality	Ginger
	Calm, steady outlook on life	Salads
	Routine-based lifestyle	Spicy Indian dishes
Pitta type	Medium-proportioned body frame	Basmati rice
	Medium-sized shoulders and hips	Milk, butter, ghee
	Fair-colored skin	Coconut, mangoes, melons
	Sun-sensitive skin	Mushrooms, peas, cabbage
	Red, blond or light brown hair	Mung beans, tofu
	Hazel or blue eyes	Turkey, chicken and shrimp
	Sleeps easily	Cinnamon, turmeric, saffron
	Practical and efficient	Vegetarian and salads
	Good organization skills	Vegetarian Indian dishes
Vata type	Small frame that is either very short or very tall	White rice
	Narrow shoulders and hips	Warm milk
	Dark-colored skin	Figs, melons, mangoes
	Dryness of skin	Cooked vegetables
	Hair prone to dandruff	Mung beans, tofu
	Gray or black eyes	Sesame oil
	Light sleeper	Chicken, turkey, seafood
	Love of constant stimulation	Ginger, cardamom, basil
	Original thinker	Thick Indian curries

Earth

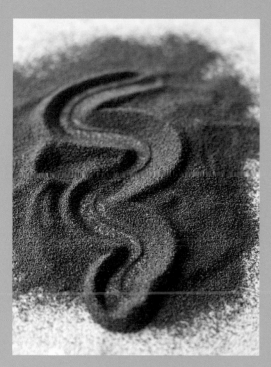

The element of Earth represents the ground on which we walk and the produce that is grown within the soil. In life, it also represents the food that we consume. It is important for us to reconnect with the cycles of nature and to eat food that is as pure as possible. Eating overly processed food and the flesh of animals suffering from environmental pollution can lead to indigestion and ultimately disease. The key message is that we should not go too far from nature otherwise we may move too far away from being healthy.

It is strongly advised that a person should eat what is known as "satvic" or "sattwic" foods, which are fresh and or organic fruit, vegetables and nuts. Ghee, or clarified butter, is also a satvic food – it is considered a tonic for the system and a good source of easy to digest fat, which can help stimulate the digestion. It is believed that satvic food improves not only the body but the mind as well. Eating fresh or freshly cooked food can help digestion and improve a person's emotional health. Overprocessed or canned food can deplete a person's energy, dull the senses and increase toxins in the body. To enhance the healing power of the food, it is important that the meal is prepared with care and feelings of love and kindness, and that the meal is eaten in relaxed surroundings.

Air

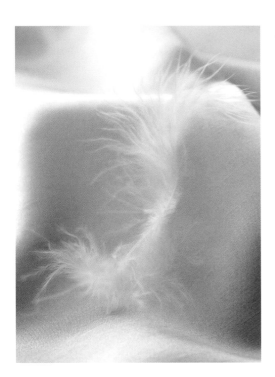

Air is a restless element that is filled with movement and a sense of constant change. It represents the stimulation of the mind and nervous system. If there is too much Air in a body's system, a person may suffer from flatulence and bloating or dryness of the skin. If there is too little air, disease may become present. Without food, a body can stay alive for some weeks. Without water, it may stay alive for a few days. However, without air, a person will only survive for a minute or two.

The air we breathe has many functions in the body including bringing oxygen into the system. According to Ayurvedic beliefs, improper breathing can lead to many health disturbances in the body. When the intake of oxygen is restricted, the body's immune system can become compromised, as improper breathing decreases blood circulation, which in turn slows down the removal of the body's waste products, such as carbon dioxide.

Such problems can be corrected by a breathing technique called pranayama, which means the control of breath or "prana" – the vital life force in the body. This ancient yogic technique is very simple and requires that you become aware of your breath. Does it sound ragged? Does it feel as if the air is only moving into the top of your lungs? If so, this may be an indication that you are feeling stressed or overly tired.

Before sitting down to a meal, practice pranayama for a few minutes as it will relax your body, release some of the stress of the day and help your digestion. When you are feeling relaxed, you will be able to appreciate your food much more, having the time to savor the tastes and textures. Once you feel relaxed and can take your time over your meal, the experience will also nurture your soul rather than giving nourishment solely to your body.

A very simplified version of a pranayama exercise is to passively observe your breathing and to imagine that the air is moving deeply through you, helping you relax. To start, imagine that the air is going into the bottom of your lungs. If you feel tension in that area, consciously relax your shoulders and chest. Then imagine that your breath is flowing into your diaphragm, solar plexus or stomach, relaxing each part of the body where you feel tension. You can continue the exercise for the rest of your body.

If you are interested in learning more about pranayama, you may wish to contact your local yoga school.

Fire

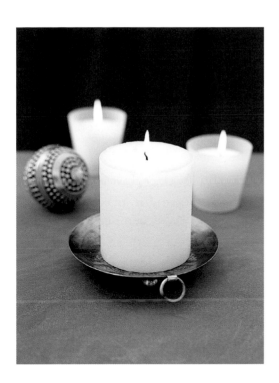

The element of Fire is an amazing one. In the universe, the sun provides the heat that encourages life on our planet. In the kitchen, fire has the ability to transform raw ingredients into the most delicious dishes. In the body, it can be seen as the digestive "fire" (*agni*) that helps break down the food we eat so that our bodies can process the nutrients and eliminate the waste. Too little digestive fire can lead to poor digestion and the build-up of toxins in the body. To much fire and food will be poorly assimilated by the body. Spices and herbs can be used in cooking to help stimulate digestive fire. In Ayurvedic medicine, it is believed that certain spices would be best suited to particular *prakruti* or constitution: kapha types may find ginger very useful, while pitta types will respond well to mint and vata types will appreciate the taste of turmeric.

Fire keeps the body physiologically active and drives all the biochemical reactions that occur in the body. The proper level of heat can have significant healing properties. In particular, heat can help improve circulation to damaged parts of the body and heighten the body's ability to heal and remove acidic waste from the area. A short burst of higher temperature can also help destroy a virus or other disease.

One important way to help stoke the fire in the body is to exercise because this form of activity can help increase various positive metabolic reactions in the body. Whenever there is more blood flow, there is a greater supply of nutrients and more efficient removal of waste and toxins. All movement in the body accelerates blood flow. Lack of exercise may lead to a deficiency in heat, which in turn leads to poor circulation and healing.

One of the most effective forms of exercise is yoga, which helps produce the heat that drives the flow of blood. It is a holistic or complete form of exercise that not only stimulates all parts of the body but also helps to connect the mind and the body. The daily practice of yoga assists the mind and body to work efficiently together. It is like daily army training, where the soldiers and their commander form a bond that leads to unquestioning obedience from the soldiers once a command is given. Similarly, yoga strengthens the connection between the body and the mind so that when the mind gives a command during an emergency the body will unfailingly answer. This is imperative for the effective healing of the body.

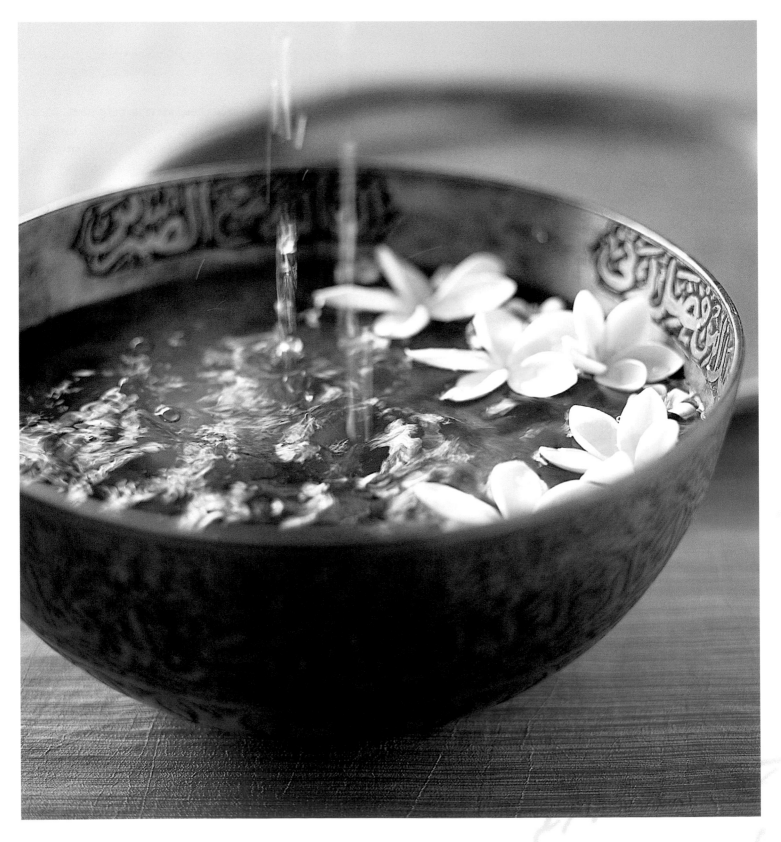

Water

Water is the most abundant element in our world and in our body. Approximately 72 percent of our body is fluid. These bodily fluids, which include our blood and digestive juices, serve many purposes, such as helping to circulate nutrients and hormones, dispose wastes and distribute heat. These fluids are the vital medium within which chemical reactions occur in the body.

The drinking of pure or filtered water is one of the most logical, natural and simple "medicines" for helping relieve the effect of disease. Many people focus on giving their bodies minute traces of vitamins, minerals, enzymes and hormones and obsessively calculate their intake of carbohydrates, proteins and fats, but forget that water is probably the safest supplement we can use everyday. Water is the major ingredient craved by our bodies.

Nevertheless, it is important that the water is pure and filtered. The regular intake of polluted water can seriously undermine your immune system. There are also some sensible rules about when and how to drink water. If your digestion is generally poor, Ayurvedic practitioners believe that it may be a good idea to reduce the amount of water taken at mealtimes. Consider drinking water half an hour before a meal and about an hour after it. This will give your own gastric juices a chance to digest the food without being watered down.

One particular Ayurvedic constitution should take particular note concerning their water intake. Kapha types, who are a combination of the elements of Water and Earth, should consider drinking their water slightly warmed. This is because the element of Water is already prominent in their constitutional makeup and if they drink too much cold water, they may find that they feel waterlogged and sluggish. It is suggested that kapha types drink a glass of warm water with a squeeze of lemon or a slice of raw ginger half an hour before their meal, as this will help stimulate their digestion.

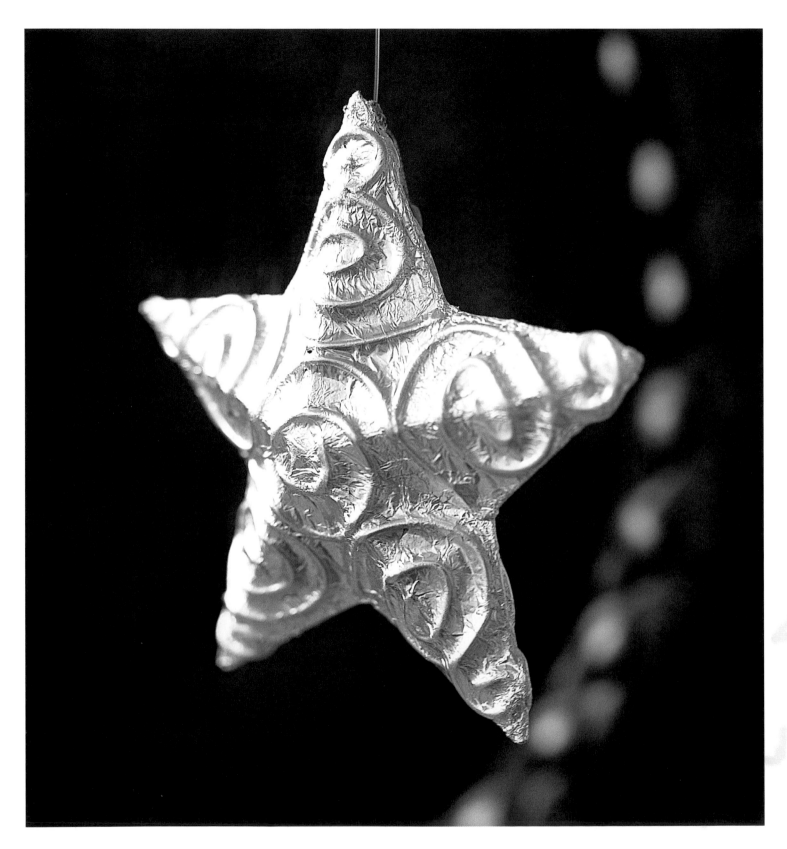

Space

The most fundamental element in the Ayurvedic system is Space or Ether, which is basically the pervasive stillness of the universe. It is believed that Space was the very first element and that everything in the cosmos is encompassed by it. The other four elements of Earth, Fire, Water and Air are manifested within Space and act as a balance.

In Ayurvedic medicine, the element of Space is represented within the body by the organs that provide voids to be filled, such as the lungs and stomach. One rule of thumb that Ayurvedic practitioners advise concerning the digestion of food is to leave the stomach feeling about two-thirds full, allowing some space for Fire, or the digestive juices, to work in utilizing the Earth and Water – the food and drink taken during the meal.

If there is no space left in the stomach, the transformations required between the Earth, Water and Fire could be undermined. Space, or the void within the organs and even the cells of the body, is as important as the actual matter of the body, as this void allows for functions to occur properly and efficiently within the body without constriction.

Space is also an exceedingly useful element to remember in our everyday lives. When stressed, we often comment that we need some "space" to think. We also need the "space" to feel relaxed. Ayurvedic practitioners strongly advise that a person must feel relaxed before they are able to both enjoy and digest a meal. In Ayurveda, there is a great understanding of the need for balance between the elements and the aspects of one's life. Accordingly, the harder you work, the more relaxation you must schedule in your life as a balance.

In our eating habits, it may be a good idea to introduce a fast day to balance the amount of matter (food and drink) that is introduced into our bodies. Fasting helps to divert the energy of the body towards the removal of waste from the body.

Kapha types benefit the most from fasting and do not feel too distressed with this process, as they tend to store more energy than they need. On the other hand, vata types usually find fasting highly problematic and should not force themselves to do so. Their constitutions tend not to store very much energy and they may feel dizzy or faint soon after missing a meal.

Ingredients and Spices

Many of the ingredients and spices that follow are found in well-stocked supermarkets. The others are carried in shops specializing in South Asian foods.

Ingredients

Basmati rice This long-grain rice, the most commonly eaten type in India, has a wonderful fragrance when cooked and complements all Indian food. When properly cooked, the grains remain separate, rather than stick together.

Chickpea flour Rich in protein and dietary fiber, this fine yellow flour is made by finely grinding dried chickpea lentils. Also known as garbanzo bean flour, *besan* or gram flour, it is used in many Indian dishes, both sweet and savory. The flour has a slightly nutty flavor and is often used as an ingredient in batters, pastries and doughs.

Chilies Though Indian cooks use many chili varieties, the recipes in this book call for primarily two types of fresh chilies: mild long green chilies, about $4^1/2$ inches (11.5 cm) long, and hot small red serrano or bird's-eye chilies about $1^1/2$ inches (4 cm) long. Because the green chilies are mild, removing the seeds will not markedly affect their heat. If you wish to temper the heat of the fresh red chilies, remove their seeds before using. Two types of whole dried chilies are called for – everyday dried red chilies and Kashmiri chilies. The latter are a particularly bright red and have a slightly sweet flavor. Look for good-quality dried chilies and do not split them to remove their seeds. If you prefer less heat, simply decrease the number of chilies used. Chili powder, made by grinding dried chilies, is used as well. Make sure you purchase a pure chili powder, and not a compound chili powder that includes other herbs and spices.

Cilantro (fresh coriander) This pungently flavored herb is used throughout India and is generally added just before serving to ensure its flavor is retained. It is sold in bunches and has dark green serrated leaves on thin stems. Chop the leaves and some of the stems when a recipe calls for chopped cilantro, as the stems also add flavor. If a recipe calls for 1 bunch fresh cilantro, use the leaves, stems and roots, if attached, unless otherwise indicated.

Coconut milk, coconut cream, desiccated coconut Coconut milk is produced by pulverizing coconut meat with water and then draining and squeezing the mixture to extract the liquid. As the milk sits, the fat rises to the surface. This fat is skimmed off and sold separately as coconut cream. The cream is much thicker and richer than the milk. Coconut milk and coconut cream are sold in cans. (Do not purchase sweetened cream of coconut, which is used in bar drinks.) If a recipe calls for coconut milk, shake the can before opening, or stir after opening. Desiccated coconut, also known as unsweetened dried shredded coconut, is finely ground dried coconut meat, and is typically sold in plastic bags.

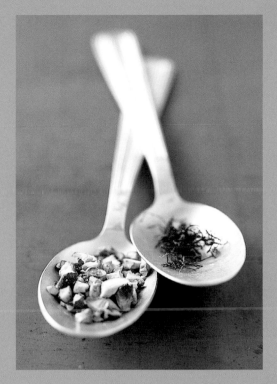

Curry leaves Native to India and Sri Lanka, curry leaves are predominantly used in southern India. Also known as karhi patta, they have a strong savory flavor with a hint of citrus. The shiny, soft dark green leaves grow on a small tree and measure roughly half the length of an index finger. Curry leaves are used in saucy dishes, spice mixes, marinades and soups. You can use dried curry leaves as a substitute, using the same number called for in the recipe.

Garlic Used throughout India except by the Hindu Brahmins and Jains, garlic is as important as onions in many Indian savory dishes. If you are cooking several recipes that call for garlic, you may want to peel a handful or so of cloves and process them in a food processor with enough sunflower, canola or other mild vegetable oil to make a paste. Keep in an airtight container in the refrigerator for up to 3 days. Substitute 1 teaspoon of this crushed garlic for 1 teaspoon minced garlic or 1 garlic clove.

Ginger, fresh Another ingredient that is ubiquitous to Indian cuisine, ginger is a rhizome with a pungent aroma and warm to hot flavor. To use fresh ginger in cooking, peel the ginger and grate on the fine rasps of a grater. If you are cooking several recipes that call for ginger, scrub the ginger to remove any dirt, coarsely chop and then process in a food processor with sunflower, canola or other mild vegetable oil to make a paste. Keep in an airtight container in the refrigerator for up to 3 days. Substitute 1 teaspoon of this crushed ginger for 1 teaspoon grated fresh ginger. The rhizome is also dried to produce ground ginger, a common Indian spice.

Indian bay leaf Despite their name, Indian bay leaves come from the cassia tree. They are larger and have a slightly sweeter flavor than European bay, though the latter can be substituted if Indian bay is unavailable.

Jaggery Made from dehydrated sugarcane juice, this sticky sweetener has a flavor resembling dark brown sugar and molasses. Dark brown sugar may be substituted, although the flavor will not be the same.

Lentils and chickpeas Two types of lentils most often used in this book are **black lentils**, also known as urad dal and black gram, and **split yellow lentils**, also known as toor dal, toovar dal, tour dal, arhar dal and pigeon peas. Black lentils are used both whole with hulls intact and hulled and split. The latter are known as split white lentils or white urad. Both black and yellow lentils are quite small in comparison with other lentils and cook faster as well, with the split lentils quickly becoming mushy. Black lentils are used in vegetable dishes, and are often roasted to add a nutty flavor. They are also ground into flour, which is combined with rice flour in dosa (page 85). Split yellow lentils are commonly used in vegetarian dishes and soups. **Red lentils** are used to a lesser degree than black or yellow lentils. Their red-orange color fades to yellow when cooked. **Chickpea lentils**, also known as garbanzo beans or Bengal gram, are used whole or split. They have a mild, slightly sweet flavor and become mushy when cooked. **Roasted split chickpeas** do not need cooking and are used in chutneys (page 112).

Mango This popular tropical fruit is used both unripe and ripe. Green mangoes are made into pickles and chutneys and are used to add tartness to savory dishes. The sweet, juicy ripe fruits are enjoyed raw or made into ice cream.

Mint The fresh leaves of this favorite herb have a clean, refreshing taste that is appreciated in many Indian dishes, including biryani, various meat and chicken preparations, raitas and homemade drinks, and the leaves are used for making hot tea. The fresh leaves are added at the end of cooking to preserve flavor.

Okra Also known as lady finger, this elegant-looking member of the mallow family is a common ingredient in Indian cooking. Okra pods exude a gelatinous juice that some people dislike, although cooks often add them to a dish for that very property, relying on the viscous substance to thicken the sauce. Okra is either cooked slowly over low heat until quite soft or quickly fried or deep-fried over high heat. Both methods ensure the pods keep their shape.

Semolina Ground from the endosperm of durum wheat, semolina has a bland flavor and slightly coarse texture. Fine semolina is used in this book. Semolina, both coarse and fine, is used in Indian sweets and some breads. It is also used as a binding agent in place of bread crumbs.

Sesame seeds These tiny seeds are harvested from a herb that grows in India and other parts of Asia. Whole or ground white sesame seeds are used in savory Indian dishes, breads and many sweets. Sometimes the seeds are toasted to heighten their nutty flavor.

Tamarind concentrate Also called tamarind paste, this concentrate is made from the pulp and seeds of the pod of the tamarind tree. It is spooned directly from the jar without the need for any of the preparation that the blocks of compressed tamarind pulp require. It adds a tart, fruity flavor to savory dishes.

Vegetable oil and unsalted butter Some of the recipes in this book call for a mixture of vegetable oil and butter. The combination has two advantages: you can heat it over relatively high heat without it beginning to smoke and it delivers good flavor. If you prefer, you can choose to use only oil and no butter. Select a monosaturated oil, such as sunflower, canola or safflower. **Mustard oil**, pressed from mustard seeds, is a pantry staple in northern and northwestern India, where it is used for pickles and for frying.

Yogurt The best yogurt to use for the recipes in this book is a thick plain (natural) yogurt made from whole (full cream) milk. Look for yogurt labeled "continental" or "Greek style" for the best consistency and flavor.

Clockwise from left: okra, fresh curry leaves, semolina, asafetida, urad dal, tamarind, jaggery, split yellow lentils, green chili, besan flour (center).

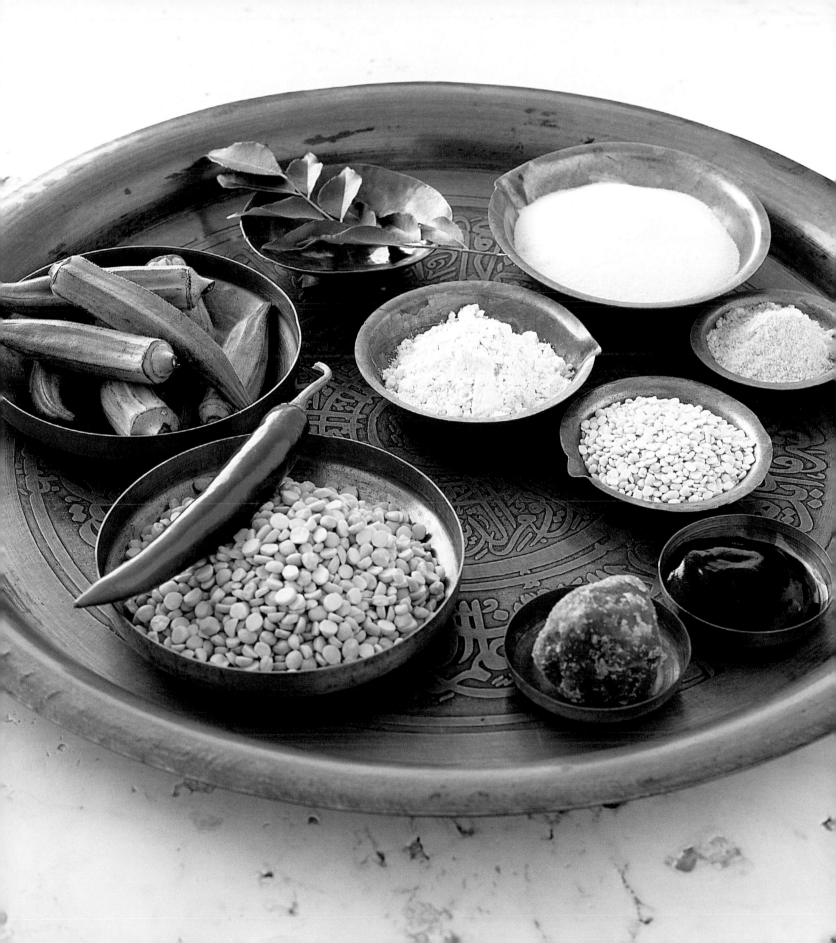

Spices

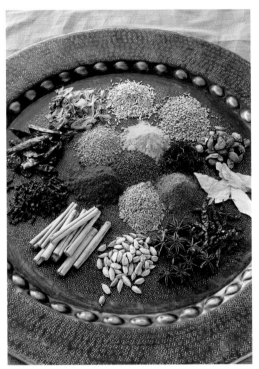

Outside, clockwise from left: cloves, dried Kashmiri chilies, blade mace, green fennel seeds, fenugreek seeds, black cardomom pods, Indian bay leaves, dried chillies, star anise, green cardomom pods, cinnamon sticks. Inside, clockwise from left: paprika, ajwain seeds, turmeric, saffron threads, chili powder, cumin seeds, black mustard seeds (center).

Aniseed Also known as anise seed, these greenish-brown seeds come from a small annual plant that is a member of the parsley family. The leaves and seed have a distinctive, sweet licorice flavor.

Asafetida Grinding the dried resinous gum extracted from roots of plants native to India and Iran produces this foul-smelling yellow powder. Its unappealing aroma disappears when it is added in small amounts to food, imparting a mild onion or garlic flavor – a fact that caught the attention of the Hindu Brahmins and Jains, whose diets do not allow the use of either popular seasoning. It is also believed to prevent the gastric distress associated with eating lentils and beans along with other foods high in fiber.

Cardamom pods Two types of cardamom are used in this book. **Whole green cardamom pods** are filled with fragrant, tiny black seeds. For the best flavor, grind just before using. In this book, pods are usually ground whole. You can also buy preground cardamom seeds. The flavor of the ground seeds is not as intense as when you grind the whole pods yourself, so you may need to increase the amount you use slightly. Green cardamom is a key ingredient in garam masala and many other spice mixes, and is used in numerous savory and sweet dishes. **Brown cardamom pods**, also called black cardamom, conceal smoky-flavored, tiny seeds. These pods are used in savory dishes and are a vital ingredient in many meat dishes.

Cinnamon sticks Also known as cinnamon quills, these hard sticks consist of rolled and layered pieces of bark from the cinnamon tree. Cinnamon sticks commonly available for cooking are 3–4 inches (7.5–10 cm) long. Many stores sell cassia sticks labeled as cinnamon. Cassia sticks, also dried bark, look similar but have a more intense fragrance. Either can be used in these recipes.

Cloves These are the dried buds of a tree that grows in Southeast Asia and the West Indies. Cloves are a key ingredient in garam masala and many other spice mixes, and are also added to rice dishes, meat dishes and sweets, where they contribute a sharp, sweet flavor.

Coriander seeds These seeds, which are harvested from the plant that provides fresh cilantro (fresh coriander), are usually dry-roasted in a frying pan and then ground and used alone or as part of a spice mix. Freshly ground coriander seeds have a lemony, herbaceous fragrance.

Cumin seeds Small, caraway shaped and aromatic, these seeds are from a plant in the parsley family. Briefly dry-roasting them brings out their flavor, which is earthy, pungent and a little bitter. Used whole or ground, cumin seeds are a common ingredient in spice mixes and in many savory dishes and raitas. Black cumin seeds are slightly less bitter than their light-colored cousins.

Fennel seeds This spice, used whole or ground, contributes an anisey flavor to meat dishes, vegetable dishes, desserts, pickles and chutneys. It is sometimes added to garam masala.

Fenugreek seeds Whole or ground fenugreek seeds are used. The rectangular seeds, roasted to bring out their nutty flavor, are added to spice mixes, breads, chutneys and lentil dishes.

Mustard seeds Black and brown mustard seeds look almost identical, but are different species. The brown seeds have only about 70 percent of the pungency of the black seeds. Either type can be used in the recipes in this book. The seeds are always crackled in hot oil for a brief time to release their pungent flavor. See the vegetable oil and unsalted butter entry under Ingredients for information on mustard oil.

Nutmeg and mace The hard, light brown seed of a tree, **nutmeg** is sold whole, for grating fresh, or ground and is commonly teamed with sweet foods. In India, it is also an ingredient in some spice mixes for savory dishes. Its mild, sweet flavor complements both white and red meats and is thought to help tenderize them. The red coating of the nutmeg seed, **mace** has a more pungent flavor than nutmeg and enhances savory dishes. Blade mace is the whole coating, which has been removed from the nutmeg and dried; it has a coarse, netted appearance. The spice is also sold ground. Mace goes well in rice dishes and seafood dishes.

Paprika This bright red spice is made by finely grinding dried red peppers. It adds flavor and color to many savory dishes and is sold in a variety of heat levels. Mild paprika, with the flavor of bell pepper (capsicum), is used in this book.

Peppercorns Sometimes called the King of Spices, peppercorns are featured extensively in Indian cooking. Use black peppercorns and always grind them just before adding to a dish to ensure the best aroma and flavor.

Saffron threads If peppercorns are the King of Spices, then saffron is the ruling queen. Saffron threads are the dried stigmas from a variety of crocus, each blossom of which produces only three stigmas. Harvesting saffron is labor-intensive, making it the most costly spice in the world. Saffron threads are generally soaked in warm liquid to release their intense gold-yellow color and pungent, earthy aroma and flavor.

Star anise This spice is the dried star-shaped pod from a variety of evergreen magnolia tree. Each point of the 8-point star contains a tiny seed. Commonly used in Chinese cooking, star anise also makes an appearance in Indian foods. Its flavor is similar to that of aniseed, but has more depth of flavor and sweetness.

Turmeric An essential ingredient for the Indian pantry, turmeric is used in most savory dishes to lend a deep gold color and sharp and sometimes bitter flavor. It also helps to amalgamate the flavors of other spices. Derived from the root of a tropical plant, turmeric is generally dried and then ground.

Step-by-step Techniques

Step-by-step
Nilgiri's garam masala

**1 cinnamon stick, 4 inches (10 cm)
long, broken into small pieces
1 tablespoon green cardamom pods
3 brown cardamom pods
1 tablespoon whole cloves
1 tablespoon blade mace
1 tablespoon black peppercorns
1 tablespoon fennel seeds
3 Indian bay leaves, torn into quarters
1 teaspoon freshly grated nutmeg**

1. Heat a small frying pan or saucepan over low heat. One at a time, dry-roast cinnamon, cardamom, cloves, mace, peppercorns, fennel seeds and bay leaves until fragrant and only lightly colored. This should take 2–3 minutes for each spice. Make sure heat is not too intense, or spices may brown too much or even burn.
2. As each spice is roasted, place in a bowl. Allow roasted spices to cool to room temperature. Add nutmeg and mix thoroughly. Transfer to a jar or other airtight container and store in the refrigerator for up to 1 year.
3. Just before using garam masala, grind to a fine powder in a spice grinder.

Makes about ⅓ cup

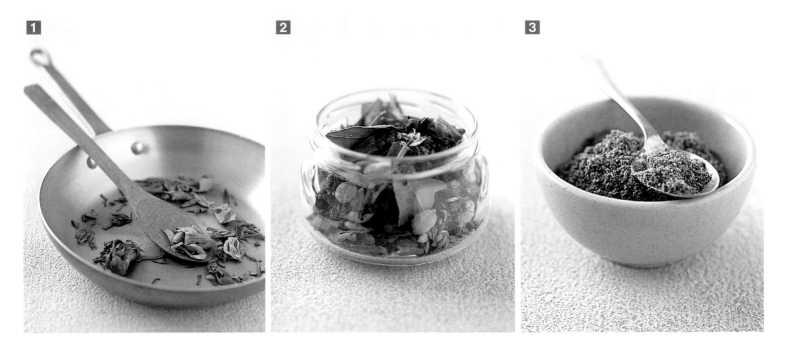

Step-by-step
Cooking onions

**¹/₂ cup (4 fl oz/125 ml) vegetable oil
or equal parts vegetable oil and
melted unsalted butter
3 yellow (brown) onions, halved and
thinly sliced or chopped
1 teaspoon salt**

Cooking onions correctly is an important step in making many Indian dishes, and the process must not be rushed, or the onions will burn. The quantities given here are similar to those found in many recipes in this book. You can use a ratio of half oil to half unsalted butter, a combination that allows you to heat the fat without fear of it smoking and also delivers good flavor. Alternatively, you can use only oil.

1. In a large, heavy-bottomed saucepan, heat oil or oil and butter over medium–low heat. Do not overheat, or butter will burn and taint onions. Add onions and salt to pan. Salt helps onions to brown evenly and adds flavor.
2. Cook uncovered, stirring occasionally, until onions are dark golden brown, 20–25 minutes. Onions around edge of pan will begin to color; stirring helps to distribute heat and ensures even browning.

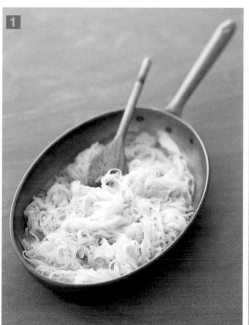
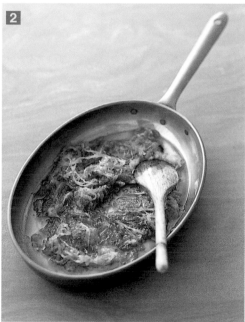

Spice Mixes

North
Vari masala

1¹/₂ oz (45 g) dried red chilies
1 tablespoon coriander seeds
3 brown cardamom pods
2 whole cloves
¹/₂ teaspoon cumin seeds
¹/₂-inch (12-mm) piece cinnamon stick
Pinch saffron threads
2 teaspoons ground ginger
Pinch powdered asafetida

1. Heat a small, nonstick frying pan over low heat. Dry-roast chilies until fragrant, 4–5 minutes. Transfer to a bowl. Dry-roast coriander, cardamom, cloves, cumin and cinnamon together until fragrant and only lightly colored, 4–5 minutes. Make sure heat is not too intense, or spices may brown too much or even burn. Remove from heat and set aside to cool slightly.
2. Place roasted chilies, coriander, cardamom, cloves, cumin, cinnamon and saffron in a spice grinder and grind to a fine powder. Transfer to a bowl and stir in ginger and asafetida.
3. Transfer to an airtight container. Store in refrigerator for up to 6 months.

Makes ¹/₂ cup

South
Coondapour masala

1 teaspoon vegetable oil
10 dried Kashmiri red chilies, broken into small pieces
2 tablespoons coriander seeds
1 teaspoon cumin seeds
1 teaspoon black peppercorns
¹/₄ teaspoon fenugreek seeds
¹/₄ teaspoon ground turmeric
10 cloves garlic, smashed
About ¹/₄ cup (2 fl oz/60 ml) water

1. In a large, nonstick frying pan, heat oil over medium heat. Add chilies, coriander, cumin, peppercorns, fenugreek, turmeric and garlic and cook, stirring, until aromatic, 7–8 minutes. Remove from heat and set aside to cool slightly.
2. Place all cooked ingredients except garlic in a spice grinder. Grind to a fine powder. Transfer to a small food processor. Add garlic and process until combined. Add water, a little at time, adding just enough for a paste to form. Stop occasionally and scrape down sides of processor.
3. Transfer to an airtight container. Store in refrigerator for up to 6 months. Use a clean spoon each time you remove masala to prevent mold from forming.

Makes about ¹/₃ cup

East
Panch phoron

2 tablespoons cumin seeds
1 tablespoon black or brown mustard seeds
1 tablespoon fennel seeds
1 teaspoon fenugreek seeds

1. Place cumin, mustard, fennel and fenugreek seeds in a small jar. Seal and shake to combine. Keep whole spices for up to 6 months in a cool, dark place.
2. To use, grind as needed into a fine powder in a spice grinder. Or, grind entire batch, transfer to an airtight container and store in refrigerator for up to 6 months.

Makes about 2/3 cup

West
Balchao masala

4 dried red chilies, broken into small pieces
4 dried Kashmiri red chilies, broken into small pieces
Boiling water as needed
1 tablespoon coriander seeds
1 teaspoon black peppercorns
1 teaspoon salt
1 teaspoon ground turmeric
15 cloves garlic, smashed
1-inch (2.5-cm) piece fresh ginger, roughly chopped
1 tablespoon coconut vinegar (see Note)
1–2 tablespoons white vinegar

1. Place chilies in a heatproof bowl and add boiling water to cover. Set aside until chilies soften, about 1 hour. Drain, reserving soaking liquid.
2. In a spice grinder, combine coriander and peppercorns and grind to a fine powder. Transfer to a small food processor and add salt, turmeric, garlic, ginger and drained chilies. Process until finely chopped. Add coconut vinegar, white vinegar and 1 tablespoon reserved soaking liquid. Process until a fine paste forms, adding a little more soaking liquid if required.
3. Transfer to an airtight container. Masala is best made 1 day before using. Store in refrigerator for up to 6 months. Use a clean spoon each time you remove masala to prevent mold from forming.

Makes about 2/3 cup

Note: Coconut vinegar is made by fermenting coconut sap. If unavailable, increase white vinegar to 2–3 tablespoons.

Central
Salan masala

1/3 cup (1 1/2 oz/45 g) desiccated coconut
1 1/2 tablespoons sesame seeds
1 tablespoon coriander seeds
1-inch (2.5-cm) piece cinnamon stick
4 whole cloves
6 green cardamom pods
1 teaspoon cumin seeds
2 teaspoons chili powder
1 teaspoon ground turmeric

1. In a small, nonstick frying pan, dry-roast coconut and sesame seeds over medium heat, stirring, until golden, 3–4 minutes. Set aside to cool slightly and then grind in a spice grinder to a fine powder. Transfer to a bowl.
2. Add coriander, cinnamon, cloves, cardamom and cumin to same pan. Dry-roast over medium heat, stirring, until fragrant, 4–5 minutes. Set aside to cool slightly and then grind in spice grinder to a fine powder. Add to coconut mixture along with chili powder and turmeric. Stir well to combine.
3. Transfer to an airtight container. Store in refrigerator for up to 6 months. Use a clean spoon each time you remove masala to prevent mold from forming.

Makes about 2/3 cup

North India

Introduction

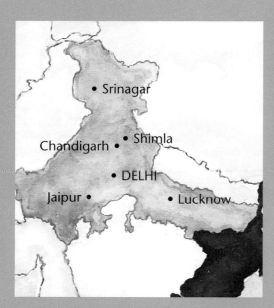

Northern India, or Uttar Bharat, is home to nearly one-fifth of the total population of India and comprises of the states of Jammu and Kashmir, Punjab, Haryana, Uttar Pradesh, Rajasthan and some parts of Gujarat. Geographically, the region is located between the Rajasthan desert to the west and the Himalayan region to the east. The climate is extreme, getting very hot in summer and very cold during the winters.

The people living in these states are predominantly farmers producing rice, especially basmati, and wheat. The grain industry is an important feature of the Punjab and Haryana agriculture. The Punjab state, in particular, is very fertile, with crops including barley, millet and sugarcane. The region, which boasts copious milk production, is also home to some famous wildlife, such as the famous Gangetic dolphin, the Indian wolf, the black-necked crane and the Himalayan tahr, which is related to the wild mountain goat.

I had the privilege of living in this part of India during my early working days. This gave me ample opportunity to learn some of the best food that this region has to offer. Northern Indian food is wrongly considered to be all kormas, full of nuts, dried fruits and cream. However, people living in North India also eat simple dishes, such as Palak Murgh (Chicken with Spinach) and Tariwale Macchi (Spicy Fish).

As food in this region predominantly revolves around wheat (roti), which is the staple meal (except for Kashmir where rice is more commonly eaten), most dishes are thicker to accompany the bread. In Kashmir, the dishes tend to be quite thin to accompany the rice. Northern India also is the home to an innovative style of cooking called Dum Pukht, which is a dish that uses the juices of meat sealed in the container as part of the Dum cooking process.

The North is also the home of the Tandoori oven and most kebabs cooked in this way have a unique taste of their own, marinated in such ingredients as ginger, lemon, garam masala and chili. Tandoori chicken is another famous dish from this region. In this chapter we have included kebabs, which can be cooked without the traditional oven. This style of Western cooking will not compromise either the taste or the flavor of the Tandoori dish.

I hope this chapter inspires you to cook a typical Northern Indian meal. These recipes still continue to inspire me after all these years!

Starters

Fried chicken
Tali murghi

1¹/₂ cups (6 oz/180 g) dried bread crumbs
¹/₂ cup (2¹/₂ oz/75 g) all-purpose (plain) flour
2 teaspoons salt
2 teaspoons chili powder
1 teaspoon coriander seeds, ground in spice grinder
1 teaspoon cumin seeds, ground in spice grinder
1 teaspoon Nilgiri's Garam Masala (page 28)
Vegetable oil for shallow frying
¹/₂ cup (4 oz/125 g) plain whole-milk yogurt
1¹/₂ lb (750 g) chicken tenderloins, cut in half lengthwise if large
Tomato, Onion and Cucumber Relish (page 56) for serving
Lemon wedges for serving

This crisp chicken is sold at many roadside eateries in New Delhi, especially near Jamma Masjid. It is usually made with bone-in chicken pieces, but here boneless chicken tenderloins, also known as chicken tenders, are used, as they are easier to eat.

1. In a large plastic bag, combine bread crumbs, flour, salt, chili powder, coriander, cumin and garam masala. Toss well to combine.
2. Pour oil to a depth of about 4 inches (10 cm) in a deep, heavy saucepan and heat to 350°F (180°C) on a deep-frying thermometer.
3. Meanwhile, put yogurt in a bowl and whisk until smooth. Dip a few pieces of chicken into yogurt, shaking off excess. Add to bread-crumb mixture and toss to coat. Place on a plate and repeat with remaining chicken, yogurt and bread-crumb mixture.
4. Carefully add a few coated chicken pieces to hot oil. Cook, turning occasionally, until golden brown, 4–5 minutes. Using tongs or a slotted spoon, transfer to a plate lined with kitchen paper.
5. Serve chicken hot with relish and lemon wedges.

Serves 4 as a starter
Serves 6–8 as a starter with 1 other starter
Serves 8–10 as a starter with all 3 starters

Fried chicken (front),
tomato, onion and cucumber relish (back left),
spiced lamb kebabs (back right)

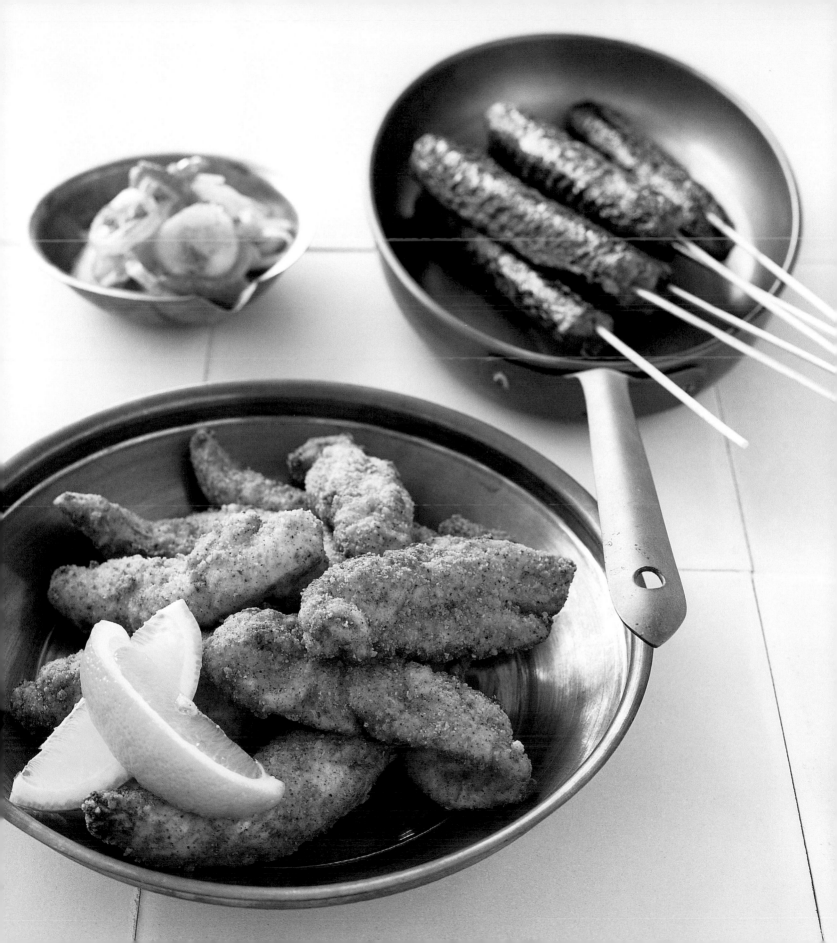

Spiced lamb kebabs
Seekh kebab

1 lb (500 g) ground (minced) lamb
4 brown cardamom pods, coarsely crushed in spice grinder
1 teaspoon ground ginger
1/2 teaspoon cumin seeds
1/4 teaspoon sugar
Tomato, Onion and Cucumber Relish (page 56) for serving

One of India's best starters, this classic kebab is usually cooked in a tandoor.

1. Soak 8 wooden skewers in cold water for 20 minutes. (Alternatively, use metal skewers.) Preheat a gas grill or prepare a charcoal grill to medium.
2. In a bowl, combine lamb, cardamom, ginger, cumin and sugar. Use your hands to mix until well combined. Divide mixture into 8 equal portions.
3. Drain skewers, and then wrap 1 portion of lamb mixture around 1 skewer, pressing it out around skewer so that it is about 6 inches (15 cm) long. Repeat with remaining lamb portions and skewers.
4. Place skewers directly over fire and cook, turning occasionally, until cooked through, 5–6 minutes.
5. Serve skewers hot with tomato relish.

Serves 4 as a starter
Serves 6–8 as a starter with 1 other starter
Serves 8–10 as a starter with all 3 starters

Lamb kebabs with onion salad
Pakay ghost ke kebab

**1 cup (8 oz/250 g) plain
whole-milk yogurt
2 tablespoons coriander seeds,
ground in spice grinder
2 tablespoons fresh lemon juice
2 tablespoons vegetable oil,
plus more for brushing
2 teaspoons grated fresh ginger
1 teaspoon salt
1/2 teaspoon chili powder
1/2 teaspoon ground turmeric
2 lb (1 kg) boneless lamb shoulder
(blade), cut into 2-inch (5-cm) cubes**

**For Onion Salad
2 yellow (brown) onions,
finely chopped
1/2 teaspoon Nilgiri's Garam Masala
(page 28)
Juice of 1/2 lemon**

I had this dish for the first time at New Delhi's Akbar Hotel in the early 1980s, and I immediately fell in love with it. It is extremely good as a cocktail snack.

1. In a glass or ceramic bowl, whisk yogurt until smooth. Add coriander, lemon juice, 2 tablespoons oil, ginger, salt, chili powder and turmeric and stir well to combine. Add lamb and stir to coat lamb evenly. Set aside for 10 minutes.
2. Transfer lamb mixture to a heavy-bottomed nonreactive saucepan. Cover and cook over low heat until meat is very tender, 45–60 minutes. Set aside to cool.
3. Soak wooden skewers in cold water for 30 minutes. (Alternatively, use metal skewers). Prepare a medium–hot fire in a charcoal grill, or preheat a gas grill on medium–high.
4. To make onion salad: In a bowl, toss together onions, garam masala and lemon juice until onions are evenly coated.
5. Drain skewers, then thread 3 or 4 pieces cooked meat onto each skewer. Brush meat lightly with oil. Place directly over fire and grill, turning once, until browned and warmed through, 2–3 minutes total.
6. Serve kebabs hot with onion salad.

Serves 4 as starter
Serves 6–8 as starter with 1 other starter
Serves 8–10 as starter with all 3 starters

Main Dishes

Chicken with apricots
Murgh khubani

1 heaping cup (6½ oz/200 g)
dried apricots
2 tablespoons vegetable oil
3 yellow (brown) onions, halved and
thinly sliced
1 teaspoon salt
2 tablespoons grated fresh ginger
1½ tablespoons minced garlic
3 fresh mild long green chilies,
slit lengthwise
3 green cardamom pods, crushed
1-inch (2.5-cm) piece cinnamon stick
1 whole chicken, 3 lb (1.5 kg), cut into
10 pieces, or 2 lb (1 kg) chicken pieces
3 ripe tomatoes, chopped
¾ cup (6 fl oz/180 ml) water
¼ teaspoon saffron threads, soaked
in 2 tablespoons warm water for
10 minutes
½ teaspoon Nilgiri's Garam Masala
(page 28)

Steamed Basmati Rice (page 141)
or Coconut Rice (page 85) and/or
Home-style Bread (page 141)
for serving
Spring Greens (page 56) for serving

In this northern version of salli murgh, a typical Parsee dish, saffron and apricots are used.

1. In a bowl, combine apricots with hot water to cover generously. Set aside for 20–30 minutes to soften. Drain and set aside.
2. Meanwhile, in a frying pan, heat oil over medium–low heat. Add onions and salt and cook uncovered, stirring occasionally, until onions are dark golden brown, 20–25 minutes.
3. Raise heat to medium, add ginger, garlic, chilies, cardamom and cinnamon and cook, stirring, until fragrant, 2–3 minutes. Raise heat to high, add chicken pieces and cook, turning occasionally, until chicken is golden brown, 3–4 minutes. Stir in tomatoes and water, reduce heat to low and cook, partially covered, until chicken is cooked through and tender, about 20 minutes.
4. Add apricots and saffron and water and stir well. Cook over low heat, stirring occasionally, for 5 minutes to blend flavors. You don't want apricots to become too soft.
5. Taste and adjust seasoning with salt if necessary. Remove from heat and stir in garam masala. Serve immediately.

Serves 4–6 with rice and/or bread and Spring Greens
Serves 6–8 with rice and/or bread, Spring Greens, 1 vegetarian main dish, and 1 lamb or seafood main dish

Chicken with apricots (front), coconut rice
(back left), spring greens (back right)

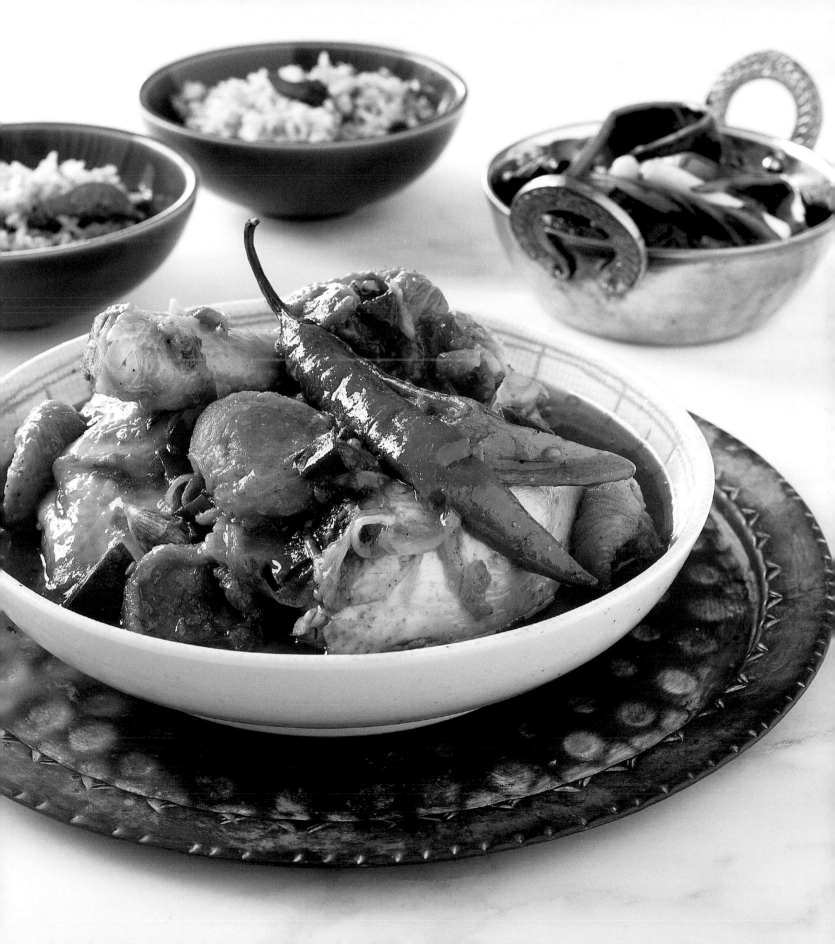

Chicken with spinach
Palak murgh

1 lb (500 g) spinach, stems removed
3 fresh mild long green chilies,
slit lengthwise
2 large yellow (brown) onions,
roughly chopped
1/2 cup (4 fl oz/125 ml) vegetable oil
1 teaspoon salt
2 1/2 tablespoons minced garlic
1 teaspoon grated fresh ginger
1/4 cup (2 fl oz/60 ml) whole milk
1 whole chicken, 3 lb (1.5 kg), cut into
10 pieces, or 2 lb (1 kg) chicken pieces
1 teaspoon Nilgiri's Garam Masala
(page 28)
1/2 teaspoon chili powder
3 ripe tomatoes, finely chopped
1/2 cup (4 fl oz/125 ml) heavy (double)
cream

Steamed Basmati Rice (page 141) or
Coconut Rice (page 85) and/or
Home-style Bread (page 141)
for serving
Spring Greens (page 56), Eggplant
with Apple (page 57) and/or Tomato,
Onion and Cucumber Relish (page 56)
for serving

You can prepare this home-style Punjabi classic with fresh fenugreek leaves in place of the spinach.

1. In a food processor, combine spinach and chilies and process until a paste forms. Transfer to a bowl and set aside. Rinse and dry processor, add onions, and process until finely ground. Remove from processor and set aside.
2. In a large, heavy-bottomed frying pan, heat oil over medium heat. Add onions and salt and cook uncovered, stirring occasionally, until lightly golden, about 15 minutes. Stir in garlic and ginger and cook, stirring, until fragrant, about 2 minutes. Stir in milk and cook for about 5 minutes longer.
3. Raise heat to high, add chicken and cook, stirring occasionally, until well browned, about 5 minutes. Stir in garam masala and chili powder and cook, stirring, until all moisture evaporates and oil separates, 5–10 minutes.
4. Stir in spinach puree and tomatoes. Cover, reduce heat to low and cook until chicken is cooked throughout and tender, 20–25 minutes. Uncover and, if liquid remains, continue to cook over medium heat until liquid evaporates.
5. Just before serving, stir in cream. Serve immediately.

Serves 4–6 with rice and/or bread and 1 or more accompaniments
Serves 6–8 with rice and/or bread, 1 or more accompaniments, 1 vegetarian main dish, and 1 lamb or seafood main dish

Chicken Dhaniwal
Dhaniwala murgh

1 whole chicken, 3 lb (1.5 kg), cut into
10 pieces, or 2 lb (1 kg) chicken pieces
2 brown cardamom pods
1/2 teaspoon ground turmeric
2 cups (16 fl oz/500 ml) water
1/3 cup (3 fl oz/90 ml) vegetable oil
2 yellow (brown) onions, halved and
thinly sliced
1 teaspoon salt
3 whole cloves
5 green cardamom pods, crushed
1-inch (2.5-cm) piece cinnamon stick
2 cups (1 lb/500 g) plain whole-milk
yogurt, whisked until smooth
1 1/2 tablespoons minced garlic
Leaves from 1 bunch fresh cilantro
(fresh coriander), chopped
1/2 teaspoon freshly ground black
pepper

Steamed Basmati Rice (page 141)
or Coconut Rice (page 85) and/or
Home-style Bread (page 141)
for serving
Spring Greens (page 56), Eggplant
with Apple (page 57) and/or Tomato,
Onion and Cucumber Relish (page 56)
for serving

I first tried this dish at the Taj Mahal Hotel in New Delhi. I knew instantly that if I ever wrote a book, this recipe would definitely be in it.

1. In a saucepan, combine chicken, brown cardamom, turmeric and water. Place over low heat, bring to a simmer and cook until chicken is almost tender, about 20 minutes. Remove chicken from stock and set aside. Strain stock through a fine-mesh sieve and reserve.
2. In a wide, heavy-bottomed saucepan, heat oil over medium–low heat. Add onions and salt and cook, stirring occasionally, until onions are dark golden brown, 20–25 minutes. Using a slotted spoon, transfer to paper towels to drain.
3. Reheat oil remaining in pan over medium heat. Add cloves, green cardamom, cinnamon, yogurt and garlic. Reduce heat to low and cook, stirring constantly, until sauce thickens, 10–15 minutes. Sauce may appear curdled at this stage, but will be fine after further cooking.
4. Add chicken to sauce in pan and cook, stirring, until sauce coats chicken. Add 1/4 cup (2 fl oz/60 ml) reserved stock and cook over low heat until chicken is cooked through and tender, about 10 minutes.
5. Stir in fried onions, cilantro and pepper. Transfer to a serving dish and serve immediately.

Serves 4–6 with rice and/or bread and 1 or more accompaniments
Serves 6–8 with rice and/or bread, 1 or more accompaniments, 1 vegetarian main dish, and 1 lamb or seafood main dish

Kashmiri lamb korma
Marzwangan korma

2 lb (1 kg) boneless lamb shoulder (blade), cut into 1-inch (2.5-cm) cubes
1/2 teaspoon ground turmeric
1 teaspoon salt
3 cups (24 fl oz/750 ml) water
1/4 cup (2 oz/60 g unsalted butter
4 green cardamom pods, crushed
6 whole cloves
2-inch (5-cm) piece cinnamon stick
3/4 teaspoon aniseed, ground in spice grinder
3/4 teaspoon chili powder
2 tablespoons paprika
1/2 teaspoon grated fresh ginger
2 teaspoons tamarind concentrate

Steamed Basmati Rice (page 141) or Coconut Rice (page 85) and/or Home-style Bread (page 141) for serving
Spring Greens (page 56), Eggplant with Apple (page 57) and/or Tomato, Onion, and Cucumber Relish (page 56) for serving

This dish, yet another Kashmiri favorite, is adapted from a recipe from the mother of my good friend Chetan Kak.

1. In a saucepan, combine lamb, turmeric, salt and water. Place over high heat and bring to a boil. Reduce heat to low and cook, uncovered, until meat is very tender, 45–60 minutes. Drain meat, reserving cooking liquid. Set meat aside.
2. In a heavy-bottomed frying pan, melt butter over medium heat. Add cardamom, cloves, cinnamon, aniseed, chili powder, paprika, ginger and tamarind. Reduce heat to low and stir until oil separates, 5–10 minutes.
3. Raise heat to high, add meat and cook, stirring, for 2–3 minutes to coat meat with seasonings. Stir in 3/4 cup (6 fl oz/180 ml) reserved stock, reduce heat to low and cook, uncovered, for 10 minutes to blend flavors. Serve immediately.

Serves 4–6 with rice and/or bread and 1 or more accompaniments
Serves 6–8 with rice and/or bread, 1 or more accompaniments, 1 vegetarian main dish, and 1 chicken or seafood main dish

Home-style bread (front), spring greens (left), Kashmiri lamb korma (back)

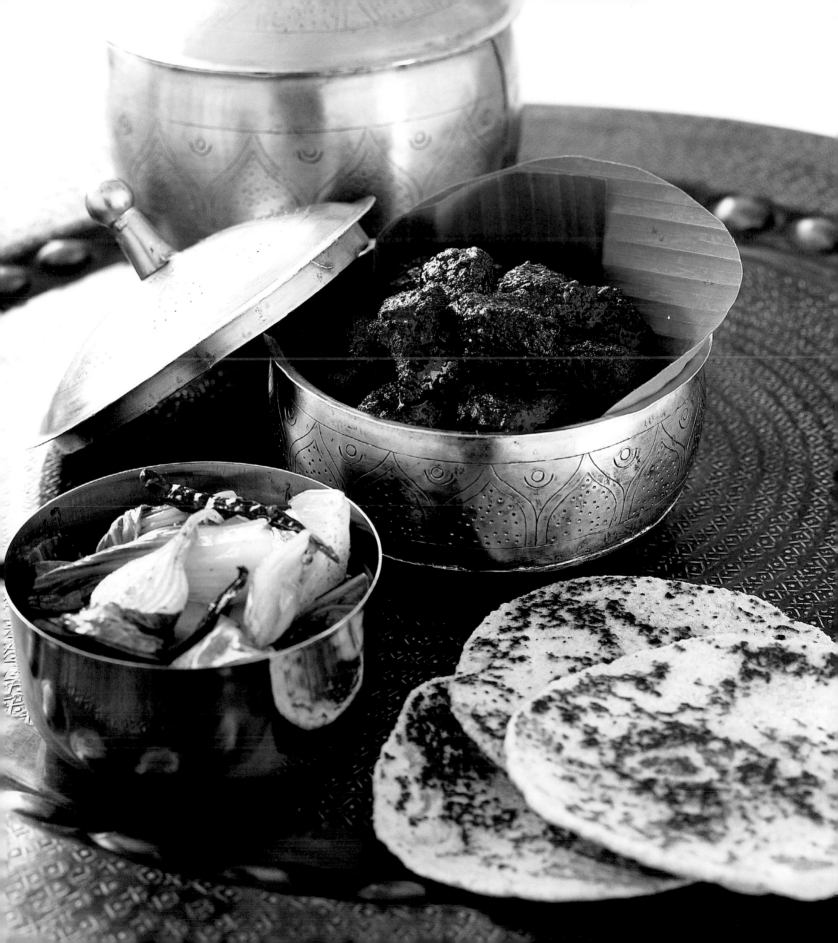

Lamb with saffron and almonds

Kalia kesar

2 tablespoons vegetable oil
3 tablespoons unsalted butter
2 yellow (brown) onions,
halved and thinly sliced
1 teaspoon salt
2 lb (1 kg) boneless lamb shoulder
(blade), cut into 2-inch (5-cm) pieces
1 tablespoon coriander seeds, ground
in spice grinder
2¹/₂ tablespoons minced garlic
¹/₄ cup (1 oz/30 g) ground almonds
³/₄ cup (6 oz/180 g) plain whole-milk
yogurt, whisked until smooth
2 cups (16 fl oz/500 ml) hot water
¹/₂ teaspoon saffron threads, soaked in
1 tablespoon hot water for 10 minutes
¹/₂ teaspoon Nilgiri's Garam Masala
(page 28)
¹/₄ cup (2 fl oz/60 ml) heavy (double)
cream

Steamed Basmati Rice (page 141) or
Coconut Rice (page 85) and/or
Home-style Bread (page 141)
for serving
Spring Greens (page 56), Eggplant
with Apple (page 57) and/or Tomato,
Onion and Cucumber Relish (page 56)
for serving

1. In a heavy-bottomed saucepan, heat oil and butter over medium-low heat. Add onions and salt and cook uncovered, stirring occasionally, until onions are dark golden brown, 20–25 minutes. Using a slotted spoon, transfer onions to a food processor. Process until finely ground. Set aside.
2. Return pan to high heat and add half of lamb to oil and butter remaining in pan. Cook, turning as needed, until browned on all sides, 2–3 minutes. Transfer lamb to plate and repeat with remaining lamb. Return lamb to pan.
3. Stir in coriander, garlic, and almonds and cook over medium heat, stirring constantly, for 2–3 minutes. Gradually stir in yogurt and then add hot water and simmer, uncovered, over low heat until meat is tender and liquid has reduced by half, about 1–1¹/₄ hours.
3. Add ground onions, saffron and water, and garam masala, stir well and cook, uncovered, over low heat until oil separates, 5–10 minutes. Stir in cream.
4. Remove from heat. Taste and adjust seasoning with salt if necessary. Transfer to a serving dish and serve immediately.

Serves 4–6 with rice and/or bread and 1 or more accompaniments
Serves 6–8 with rice and/or bread, 1 or more accompaniments, 1 vegetarian main dish, and 1 chicken or seafood main dish

Lamb with spinach
Palak maaz

1/2 cup (4 fl oz/125 ml) vegetable oil
2 lb (1 kg) boneless lamb shoulder
(blade), cut into 1-inch (2.5-cm) pieces
1/4 teaspoon powdered asafetida
1 teaspoon salt
4 whole cloves
2 teaspoons chili powder
2 teaspoons ground ginger
2 lb (1 kg) spinach, stems removed
1/2 teaspoon Nilgiri's Garam Masala
(page 28)

Steamed Basmati Rice (page 141) or
Coconut Rice (page 85) and/or
Home-style Bread (page 141)
for serving
Spring Greens (page 56), Eggplant
with Apple (page 57) and/or Tomato,
Onion and Cucumber Relish (page 56)
for serving

Here is another Kashmiri lamb dish from Chetan Kak's mother, this one distinguished by the addition of asafetida.

1. In a large, heavy bottomed saucepan, heat oil over high heat. Working in 3 or 4 batches, add lamb and cook on all sides until well browned, 3–4 minutes. As each batch is ready, transfer it to a plate.
2. Add asafetida, salt, cloves, chili powder and ginger to pan over high heat and cook, stirring, for 1 minute. Stir in spinach, cover and cook until spinach wilts, 5–8 minutes.
3. Return lamb to pan, cover and cook over medium–low heat until lamb is tender, 45–60 minutes.
4. Taste and adjust seasoning with salt if necessary. Transfer to a serving dish, sprinkle with garam masala and serve immediately.

Serves 4–6 with rice and/or bread and 1 or more accompaniments
Serves 6–8 with rice and/or bread, 1 or more accompaniments, 1 vegetarian main dish, and 1 chicken or seafood main dish

Spicy fish
Tariwale macchi

1/3 cup (3 fl oz/90 ml) vegetable oil
3 yellow (brown) onions, finely chopped
1 teaspoon salt
1 1/2 tablespoons minced garlic
1 teaspoon grated fresh ginger
4 tomatoes, finely chopped
1 teaspoon coriander seeds, ground in spice grinder
1/2 teaspoon aniseed, ground in spice grinder
1/2 teaspoon ground turmeric
1/2 teaspoon chili powder
1/2 teaspoon Nilgiri's Garam Masala (page 28)
1 cup (8 fl oz/250 ml) water
1/2 cup (4 oz/125 g) plain whole-milk yogurt, whisked until smooth
1 1/2 lb (750 g) white fish fillets such as snapper or cod, skin and bones removed, cut into serving-sized portions if large
1 tablespoon chopped fresh mint
1 tablespoon chopped fresh cilantro (fresh coriander)

Steamed Basmati Rice (page 141) or
Coconut Rice (page 85) and/or
Home-style Bread (page 141)
for serving
Spring Greens (page 56), Eggplant with Apple (page 57) and/or Tomato, Onion and Cucumber Relish (page 56)
for serving

Although this spicy dish is a traditional main dish, it also makes a good cocktail snack if you cut the fish into 1-inch (2.5-cm) pieces. You can also substitute shrimp for the fish.

1. In a wide, heavy-bottomed saucepan, heat oil over medium–low heat. Add onions and salt and cook, stirring occasionally, until onions are dark golden brown, 20–25 minutes. Raise heat to medium, add garlic and ginger and cook, stirring, for 2 minutes.
2. Add tomatoes, coriander, aniseed, turmeric, chili powder and garam masala and stir over medium heat for 2 minutes. Stir in water and yogurt.
3. Add fish to pan and spoon sauce over it. Cook over low heat uncovered, turning once, until fish is just cooked and flakes when tested with a fork, 8–10 minutes.
4. Taste and adjust seasoning with salt if necessary. Transfer to a serving dish and sprinkle with mint and cilantro. Serve immediately.

Serves 4–6 with rice and/or bread and 1 or more accompaniments
Serves 6–8 with rice and/or bread, 1 or more accompaniments, 1 vegetarian main dish, and 1 chicken or lamb main dish

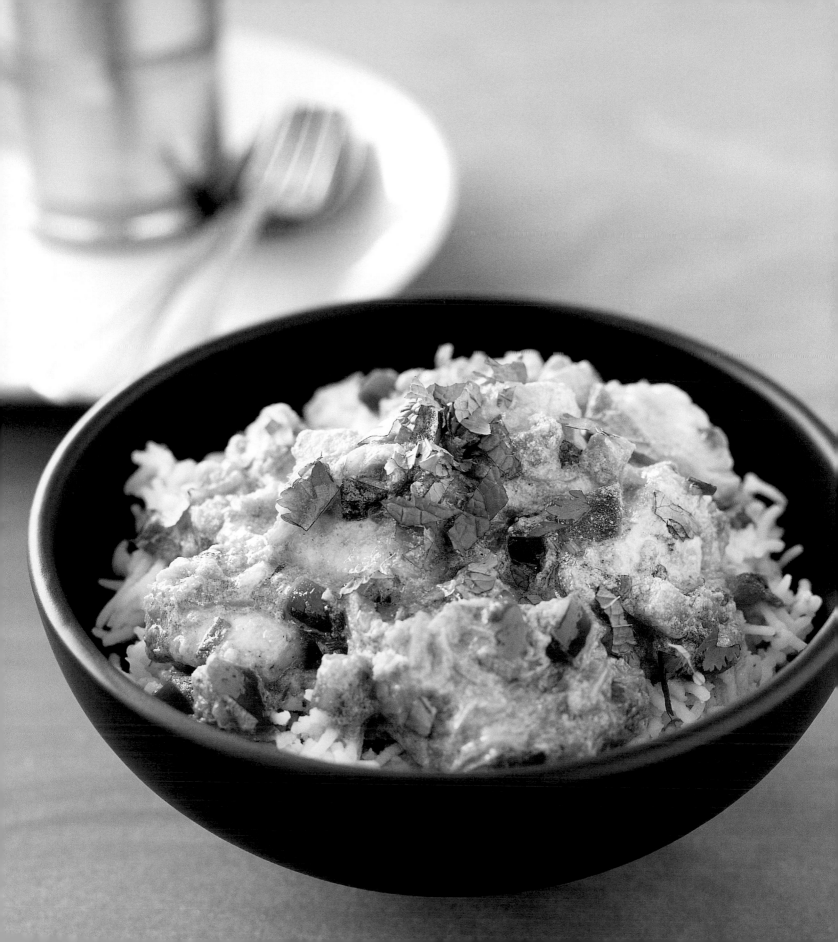

Kashmiri fish curry
Gada

1 cup (8 fl oz/250 ml) mustard oil
2 lb (1 kg) white-fleshed fish fillets such as snapper or cod, skin and bones removed, cut into serving-sized portions
2 cups (16 fl oz/500 ml) water
1 tablespoon fennel seeds, ground in spice grinder
2 teaspoons ground turmeric
2 teaspoons salt
1/2 teaspoon cumin seeds
6 black peppercorns
1 tablespoon minced garlic
2 teaspoons grated fresh ginger
1 teaspoon chili powder
1–2 teaspoons Vari Masala (page 30)

Steamed Basmati Rice (page 141) or Coconut Rice (page 85) and/or Home-style Bread (page 141) for serving
Spring Greens (page 56), Eggplant with Apple (page 57) and/or Tomato, Onion and Cucumber Relish (page 56) for serving

This is a Kashmiri Brahmin style fish using vari masala.

1. In a heavy-bottomed frying pan, heat oil over high heat. Once oil starts to smoke, reduce heat to medium–high. Working in batches, add fish and cook, turning once, until golden on both sides and almost cooked, 2–3 minutes. Remove from pan using a slotted spoon and set aside. Reserve hot oil in pan.
2. In a large frying pan, combine water, fennel, turmeric, salt, cumin, peppercorns, garlic and ginger and place over medium heat. Bring to a gentle simmer.
3. Add fish to pan and place chili powder in a little pile on top. Quickly pour 2 tablespoons of hot oil reserved from frying fish over top. Cook over low heat until fish is cooked and flakes when tested with a fork, 2–3 minutes.
4. Transfer to a serving dish and sprinkle vari masala over top. Serve immediately.

Serves 4–6 with rice and/or bread and 1 or more accompaniments
Serves 6–8 with rice and/or bread, 1 or more accompaniments, 1 vegetarian main dish, and 1 chicken or lamb main dish

Tandoori shrimp
Tandoori jhinga

2 lb (1 kg) jumbo shrimp (prawns), peeled and deveined

For Marinade
**1¹/₂ cups (12 oz/375 g) plain whole-milk yogurt
1 tablespoon fresh lemon juice
1 tablespoon grated fresh ginger
1 yellow (brown) onion, minced
2 teaspoons Nilgiri's Garam Masala (page 28)
2 teaspoons chili powder
¹/₄ cup (2 fl oz/60 ml) vegetable oil
1 teaspoon salt**

For Batter
**¹/₂ cup (4 oz/125 g) plain whole-milk yogurt
2 tablespoons heavy (double) cream
2 large eggs
¹/₂ cup (2¹/₂ oz/75 g) all-purpose (plain) flour**

**Steamed Basmati Rice (page 141) or Coconut Rice (page 85) and/or Home-style Bread (page 141) for serving
Spring Greens (page 56), Eggplant with Apple (page 57) and/or Tomato, Onion and Cucumber Relish (page 56) for serving**

Tandoori cuisine would be incomplete without this simple yet mouthwatering dish, which my friend Robert calls "tandoori jalpari" (butterfly). Here, it is cooked in a conventional oven.

1. Have shrimp ready. To make marinade: In a bowl, whisk together yogurt, lemon juice, ginger, onion, garam masala, chili powder, oil and salt until well combined.
2. Add shrimp to marinade and turn to coat shrimp well. Cover and refrigerate for 4 hours.
3. To make batter: In a wide, shallow bowl, whisk together all batter ingredients until well combined.
4. Preheat oven to 425°F (220°C/Gas 7). Line 2 rimmed baking sheets with parchment (baking) paper. Lightly oil 12 metal skewers.
5. Remove shrimp from marinade. Evenly divide shrimp among prepared skewers, threading shrimp so skewer runs the length of body. You should have about 3 shrimp on each skewer. One at a time, carefully dip skewered shrimp into batter, spooning batter over shrimp and letting any excess drip off. Place on prepared baking sheet and repeat with remaining skewered shrimp.
6. Bake until shrimp are just cooked through and batter is set, 5–6 minutes. Serve hot.

Serves 4–6 with rice and/or bread and 1 or more accompaniments
Serves 6–8 with rice and/or bread, 1 or more accompaniments, 1 vegetarian main dish, and 1 chicken or lamb main dish

Spiced spinach
Moghlai saag

1/4 cup (2 fl oz/60 ml) vegetable oil
1/4 cup (2 oz/60 g) unsalted butter
1/2 teaspoon fennel seeds
4 green cardamom pods
3 yellow (brown onions), halved and thinly sliced
1-inch (2.5-cm) piece fresh ginger, peeled and cut into thin sticks
3 lb (1.5 kg) spinach, stems removed
1 teaspoon salt
1/4 teaspoon chili powder
1/2 teaspoon Nilgiri's Garam Masala (page 28)

Steamed Basmati Rice (page 141) or Coconut Rice (page 85) and/or Home-style Bread (page 141) for serving
Spring Greens (page 56), Eggplant with Apple (page 57) and/or Tomato, Onion and Cucumber Relish (page 56) for serving

There are probably as many versions as there are cooks of this simple spinach dish. This is my favorite way to make it.

1. In a large, heavy-bottomed saucepan, heat oil and butter over medium heat. Add fennel and cardamom and cook, stirring, until fragrant, 2–3 minutes. Stir in onions and ginger, reduce heat to low, and cook uncovered, stirring occasionally, until onions are dark golden brown, 20–25 minutes.
2. Add half of spinach to pan, cover and cook until it starts to wilt, 3–5 minutes. Add remaining spinach, cover and cook, uncovering and stirring often to ensure even cooking, until all spinach is wilted, about 5 minutes longer.
3. Stir in salt, chili powder and garam masala, mixing well. Transfer to a serving dish and serve hot.

Serves 4–6 (vegetarian menu) with rice and/or bread, 1 or more accompaniments, and Red Lentil Dal (page 137)
Serves 4–6 (meat menu) with rice and/or bread, 1 or more accompaniments, and 1 chicken, meat or seafood main dish
Serves 6–8 (vegetarian menu) with rice and/or bread, 1 or more accompaniments, Red Lentil Dal (page 137), and 1 other vegetarian main dish
Serves 6–8 (meat menu) with rice and/or bread, 1 or more accompaniments, Red Lentil Dal (page 137) or 1 other vegetarian main dish, and 1 chicken, meat or seafood main dish

Eggplant with apple (front), spiced spinach (back)

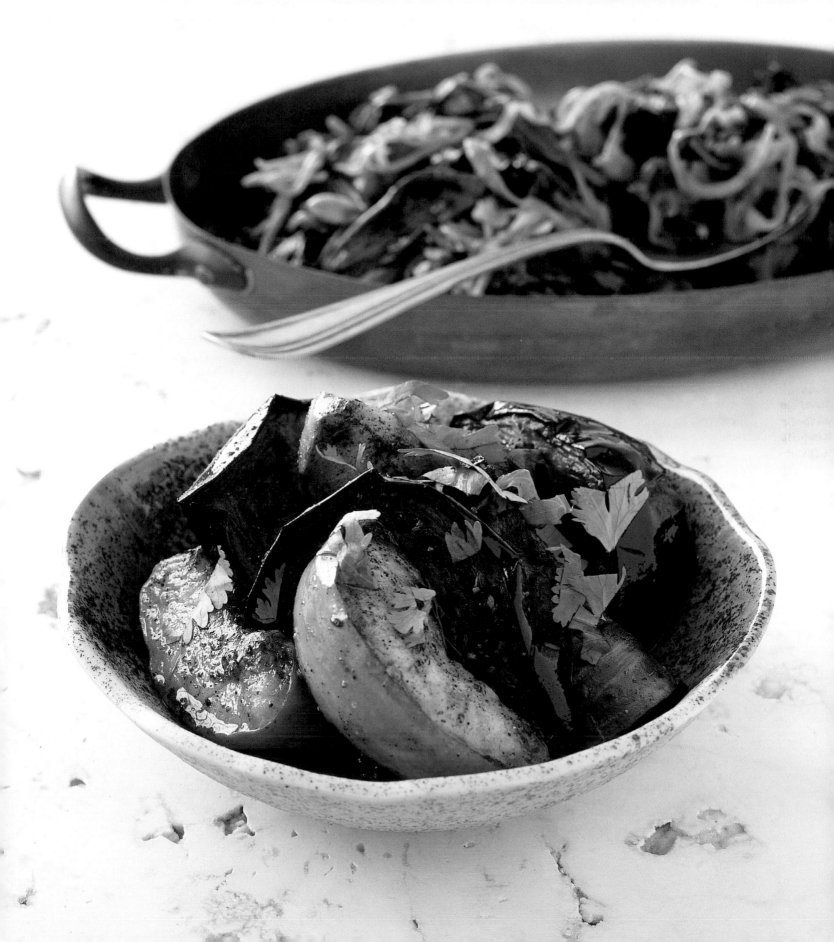

Cauliflower in spicy yogurt
Gobi dum

1/2 cup (4 fl oz/125 ml) vegetable oil
Pinch powdered asafetida
1 teaspoon cumin seeds
1 large or 2 small cauliflowers,
2 lb (1 kg) total weight, cut into small
florets with long stems attached
1 teaspoon salt
1/2 teaspoon chili powder
1-inch (2.5-cm) piece fresh ginger,
peeled and cut into thin sticks
11/2 teaspoons coriander seeds,
ground in spice grinder
1/2 teaspoon ground turmeric
1/2 teaspoon Nilgiri's Garam Masala
(page 28)
1 tablespoon fresh lemon juice
2 tablespoons plain whole-milk yogurt
2 tablespoons chopped fresh cilantro
(fresh coriander)

Steamed Basmati Rice (page 141) or
Coconut Rice (page 85) and/or
Home-style Bread (page 141)
for serving
Spring Greens (page 56), Eggplant
with Apple (page 57) and/or Tomato,
Onion, and Cucumber Relish (page 56)
for serving

Here, cauliflower florets are pot-roasted, a traditional cooking method of the North, with garam masala and other spices.

1. In a wok or deep frying pan, heat oil over medium heat. When hot, add asafetida and cumin and cook, stirring, for 20 seconds. Add cauliflower florets, cover and cook until beginning to soften, about 2 minutes.
2. Uncover and cook, stirring and tossing, for 2 minutes. Re-cover and cook until cauliflower starts to brown. Again, uncover and cook, stirring and tossing for 2 minutes, and then recover and cook for 1–2 minutes longer. At this point, cauliflower should be golden brown.
3. Reduce heat to low and add salt, chili powder, ginger, coriander, turmeric, garam masala, lemon juice and yogurt. Mix well and cook, tossing, for 2 minutes to blend flavors.
4. Transfer to a serving dish and sprinkle with cilantro. Serve immediately.

Serves 4–6 (vegetarian menu) with rice and/or bread, 1 or more accompaniments, and Red Lentil Dal (page 137)
Serves 4–6 (meat menu) with rice and/or bread, 1 or more accompaniments, and 1 chicken, meat or seafood main dish
Serves 6–8 (vegetarian menu) with rice and/or bread, 1 or more accompaniments, Red Lentil Dal (page 137) or 1 other vegetarian main dish
Serves 6–8 (meat menu) with rice and/or bread, 1 or more accompaniments, Red Lentil Dal (page 137), 1 other vegetarian main dish, and 1 chicken, meat or seafood main dish

Home-style mixed vegetables
Mili juli subza

2¹/₂ tablespoons unsalted butter
¹/₂ teaspoon cumin seeds, ground in spice grinder
¹/₂ teaspoon ground turmeric
1 yellow (brown) onion, finely chopped
1 teaspoon salt
2 teaspoons minced garlic
1 teaspoon grated fresh ginger
¹/₂ small cauliflower, cut into small florets
4 large, ripe tomatoes, chopped
3 carrots, peeled and chopped
¹/₄ cup (2 fl oz/60 ml) water
1 cup (5 oz/150 g) shelled English peas
3 fresh mild long green chilies, slit lengthwise
¹/₄ cup (¹/₃ oz/10 g) chopped fresh cilantro (fresh coriander)
1 teaspoon Nilgiri's Garam Masala (page 28)

Steamed Basmati Rice (page 141) or Coconut Rice (page 85) and/or Home-style Bread (page 141) for serving
Spring Greens (page 56), Eggplant with Apple (page 57) and/or Tomato, Onion and Cucumber Relish (page 56) for serving

This easy-to assemble dish, with its bright colors and aromatic spices, is typical of everyday cooking in the north.

1. In a saucepan, melt butter over medium heat. Add cumin and turmeric and cook, stirring, until fragrant, 2–3 minutes. Stir in onion and salt, reduce heat to medium–low and cook uncovered, stirring often, until onion is softened, 10–15 minutes. Stir in garlic and ginger and cook, stirring, for 2 minutes.
2. Add cauliflower, tomatoes, carrots and water, cover and cook until vegetables are nearly tender, about 20 minutes. Add peas, re-cover and cook until peas are tender and flavors are blended, about 10 minutes longer.
3. Remove from heat and stir in chilies and cilantro. Transfer to a serving dish and sprinkle with garam masala. Serve immediately.

Serves 4–6 (vegetarian menu) with rice and/or bread, 1 or more accompaniments, and Red Lentil Dal (page 137)
Serves 4–6 (meat menu) with rice and/or bread, 1 or more accompaniments, and 1 chicken, meat or seafood main dish
Serves 6–8 (vegetarian menu) with rice and/or bread, 1 or more accompaniments, Red Lentil Dal (page 137), and 1 other vegetarian main dish
Serves 6–8 (meat menu) with rice and/or bread, 1 or more accompaniments, Red Lentil Dal (page 137) or 1 other vegetarian main dish, and 1 chicken, meat or seafood main dish

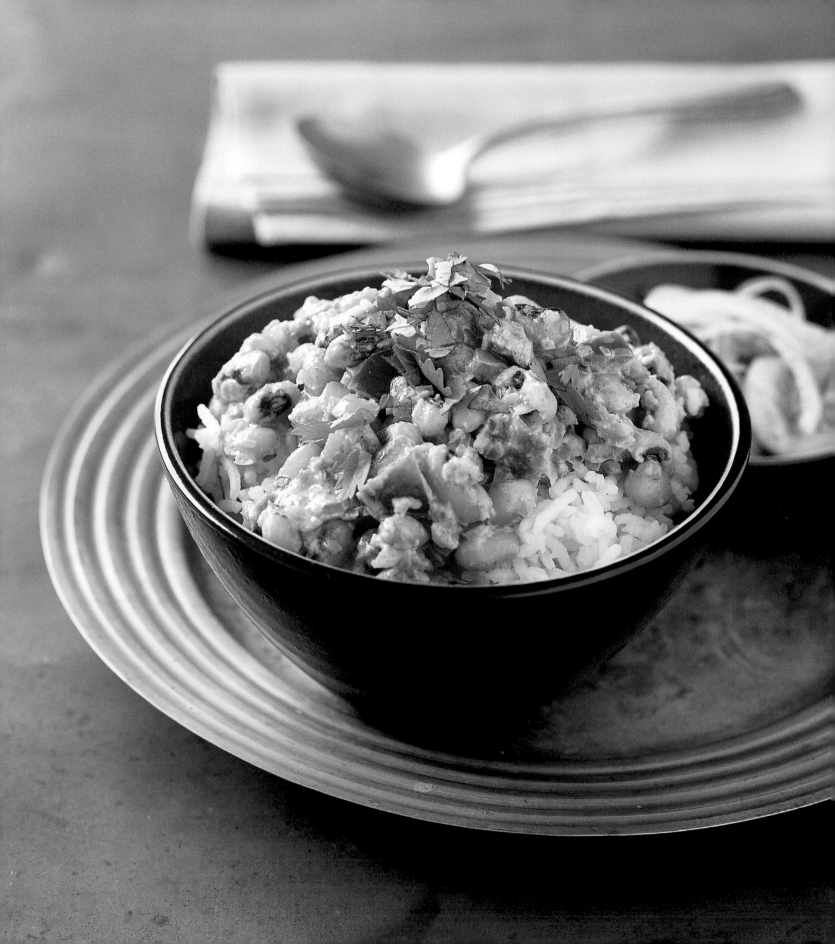

Punjabi black-eyed peas
Punjabi lobhia

1 cup (7 oz/220 g) dried black-eyed peas
1/2 teaspoon ground turmeric
1/3 cup (3 fl oz/90 ml) vegetable oil
2 yellow (brown) onions, chopped
1 teaspoon salt
1 1/2 tablespoons minced garlic
1 tablespoon grated fresh ginger
2 teaspoons coriander seeds, ground in spice grinder
1 teaspoon cumin seeds, ground in spice grinder
1/2 teaspoon chili powder
1 large, ripe tomato, chopped
1/3 cup (3 oz/90 g) plain whole-milk yogurt, whisked until smooth
2 tablespoons chopped fresh cilantro (fresh coriander)

Steamed Basmati Rice (page 141) or Coconut Rice (page 85) and/or Home-style Bread (page 141) for serving
Spring Greens (page 56), Eggplant with Apple (page 57) and/or Tomato, Onion and Cucumber Relish (page 56) for serving

When I lived in New Delhi, Sunday nights during winter were usually spent watching Hindi movies on television and eating this Punjabi dish with rice.

1. Rinse peas under cold running water until water runs clear. Place in a bowl, add water to cover generously, and set aside overnight to soak.
2. Next day, drain peas. Place in a large saucepan with turmeric and water to cover. Bring to a simmer over medium heat and cook, uncovered, until tender, 20–30 minutes. Remove from heat, drain and set peas aside.
3. In a large frying pan, heat oil over medium–low heat. Add onions and salt and cook uncovered, stirring often, until onions are softened, 10–15 minutes. Stir in garlic, ginger, coriander, cumin and chili powder and cook, stirring, until fragrant, 2–3 minutes. Stir in tomato and cook until softened, about 10 minutes.
4. Stir in yogurt, mixing well. Add cooked peas, and stir and toss until heated through. Transfer to serving dish and garnish with cilantro. Serve immediately.

Serves 4–6 (vegetarian menu) with rice and/or bread, 1 or more accompaniments, and Red Lentil Dal (page 137)
Serves 4–6 (meat menu) with rice and/or bread, 1 or more accompaniments, and 1 chicken, meat or seafood main dish
Serves 6–8 (vegetarian menu) with rice and/or bread, 1 or more accompaniments, Red Lentil Dal (page 137) or 1 other vegetarian main dish
Serves 6–8 (meat menu) with rice and/or bread, 1 or more accompaniments, Red Lentil Dal (page 137), 1 other vegetarian main dish, and 1 chicken, meat or seafood main dish

Punjabi black-eyed peas and tomato, onion and cucumber relish

Accompaniments

Spring greens
Karam ka saag

1/2 cup (4 fl oz/125 ml) mustard oil
3 dried red chilies
1/2 teaspoon chili powder
1 1/2 teaspoons coriander seeds,
ground in spice grinder
1 1/2 lb (750 g) assorted leafy greens
and other spring vegetables such as
baby spinach, bok choy and scallions
(shallots/spring onions), trimmed
and cut into 1-inch (2.5-cm) pieces
1 1/2 tablespoons minced garlic
Salt

A great accompaniment to any meal.

1. In a large saucepan, heat oil over medium–high heat. When it starts to smoke, reduce heat to medium.
2. Add chilies, chili powder, coriander and any greens with firm stems. Stir and toss for 2 minutes. Add remaining greens and garlic and cook, tossing, until leaves wilt, 1–2 minutes.
3. Season to taste with salt. Remove and discard whole chilies. Transfer to a serving dish and serve hot.

Serves 6–8

Tomato, onion and cucumber relish
Laccha

1 yellow (brown) onion, halved and
thinly sliced
2 ripe tomatoes, peeled and
thinly sliced
2 cucumbers, peeled and thinly sliced
2 tablespoons fresh lemon juice
1/2 teaspoon salt
1/4 teaspoon chili powder
Freshly ground black pepper
1/2 teaspoon cumin seeds, dry-roasted
on stove top and ground
in spice grinder

A great accompaniment to any meal.

1. In a small bowl, combine onion, tomato, cucumber, lemon juice and salt and stir to combine. Taste and adjust seasoning with salt.
2. Sprinkle chili powder, pepper and cumin over relish. Serve soon after making.

Serves 6–8

Eggplant with apple
Tsoont wasngan

4 cooking apples
2 lb (1 kg) small eggplants
(aubergines)
1 cup (8 fl oz/250 ml) mustard oil
Pinch powdered asafetida
1 teaspoon paprika
1 teaspoon salt
1/2 teaspoon ground turmeric
1/2 teaspoon chili powder
1 teaspoon cumin seeds, ground
in spice grinder
1/2 teaspoon aniseed, ground
in spice grinder
1 tablespoon chopped fresh cilantro
(fresh coriander)

A great accompaniment to any meal.

1. Core each apple and cut into 6 wedges. Trim eggplants and cut crosswise into slices 1 inch (2.5 cm) thick. If eggplants are large, cut in half lengthwise before slicing.
2. In a frying pan, heat oil over medium–high heat. When it starts to smoke, reduce heat to medium.
3. Add apple wedges and cook, turning once, until golden brown, 3–4 minutes on each side. Using a slotted spoon, transfer apples to a plate lined with paper towels.
4. Reheat oil remaining in pan over medium–high heat. Add a few eggplant slices and cook, turning once, until golden brown on both sides, 3–4 minutes on each side. Using a slotted spoon, transfer eggplant slices to a plate lined with paper towels. Repeat until all eggplant slices are browned.
5. Reheat oil over medium heat. Add asafetida, paprika, salt, turmeric, chili powder, cumin and aniseed and stir well. Add eggplant and apple pieces to pan and toss to combine and heat through. Taste and adjust seasoning with salt.
6. Transfer to serving dish and sprinkle with cilantro. Serve warm.

Serves 6–8

Desserts

Warm apple pudding
Saeb

3 lb (1.5 kg) cooking apples, cored and grated
1 tablespoon sugar
Juice of 1 lemon
²/₃ cup (5 oz/150 g) unsalted butter
2-inch (5-cm) piece cinnamon stick
5 whole cloves
²/₃ cup (5 fl oz/150 ml) condensed milk
2 tablespoons raisins
Slivered blanched almonds for garnish

1. In a bowl, combine apples, sugar and lemon juice and toss to combine. Set aside.
2. In a heavy-bottomed saucepan, melt butter over medium heat. Add cinnamon and cloves and cook, stirring, until fragrant, 2–3 minutes. Raise heat to high, add apples and cook, stirring occasionally, until apple is very soft and liquid is absorbed, 8–10 minutes.
3. Stir in condensed milk and raisins and cook, stirring, for about 5 minutes.
4. Spoon into individual bowls and top with almonds. Serve warm.

Serves 6

Pumpkin halwa
Kaddu halwa

1 pumpkin, 4 lb (2 kg), halved, seeded, peeled and chopped
1¹/₂ cups (12 oz/375 g) sugar
6¹/₂ oz (200 g) unsalted butter
1 cup (8 fl oz/250 ml) whole milk
4 green cardamom pods, crushed
1 cup (4 oz/125 g) slivered blanched almonds
¹/₂ cup (3 oz/90 g) raisins, roughly chopped
2 teaspoons rose water (optional)
Toasted desiccated coconut for serving

1. In heavy-bottomed saucepan, combine pumpkin, sugar, butter and milk and place over low heat. Cook, stirring, until sugar dissolves. Raise heat to medium–low and simmer uncovered, stirring occasionally, until pumpkin is very soft, 20–25 minutes.
2. Stir in cardamom and almonds and cook, uncovered, over low heat until mixture is quite thick, 30–40 minutes.
3. Stir in raisins and rose water if using and remove from heat. Spoon into individual bowls and top with coconut. Serve warm.

Serves 6–8

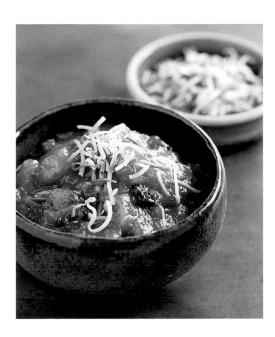

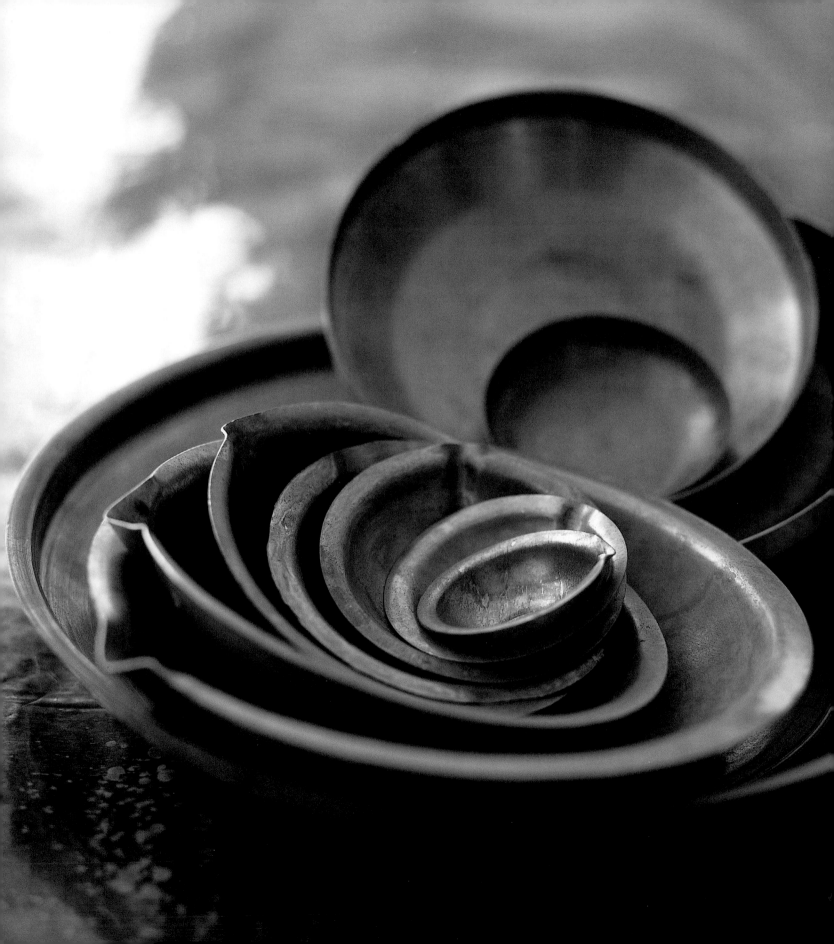

South India

Introduction

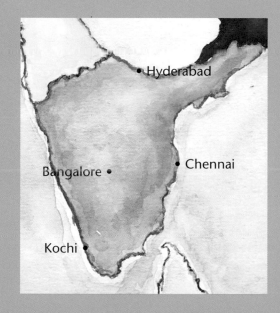

Such states as Tamilnadu, Karnataka and Kerala and the territory of Pondicherry form the Dhakishna Bharath or South Region of India. One fifth of the population of India lives in the southern states. This region geographically lies between the two famous coasts of the Indian Malabar to the west, and Koramandel and the Bay of Bengal to the east. It covers almost the entire peninsula of India.

This region is renowned for its famous temples like the Tanjore Mahabalipuram, the Madurai Meenakshi temple and the Humpe monument. The predominant religious belief in this area is a branch of Hinduism called Vaishnavism. Vaishnavaites revere Vishnu the preserver or sustainer. However, other people in this region are also Muslim and Buddhist. The largest Buddhist monastery can be found in Karnataka. Also, Kochi in Kerala has one of the oldest existing synagogues in the world called the Cochin Jewish Synagogue.

Climatic conditions in this part of India are temperate and it attracts a heavy rainfall. Many people in this part of India are farmers, like the northern Indians, but they have diversified into spices, herbs and coffee beans. Cardamom is particularly successfully cultivated in the Nilgiri Mountains. The famous Nilgiri tea is also grown in this region. Wildlife seen in this part of India includes the Nilgiri langurs (sacred monkeys) and goatlike tahrs, dolphins, catlike Malabar civets, elephants and giant squirrels.

Rice, which is the predominant grain, is cultivated in large quantities. Food from this region is spicy and hot and the sauces tend to be thin to accompany the staple diet of rice. This region's cooking, which is supposed to be the spiciest in the country, is also the birthplace of the so-called Madras Curry. The word "curry" is a corruption of the Tamil word "kari" meaning a pepper-flavored sauce.

Most dishes are cooked in earthenware pots in which they are left overnight to be consumed the following day. The belief is that rice should be made fresh and hot and the curry or kari should never be reheated. This is really the essence of cooking in the South Region of India. Another famous dish, which has its origins in this part of the country, is Neer Dosa (Rice Pancakes), which is eaten for breakfast, lunch, dinner or any time in between. Since the region has so much land girded by sea, fish is also an important ingredient for various meals, as is coconut.

I'm sure you'll enjoy cooking Southern style!

Starters

Chicken with coconut
Coondapur koli thalna

1 lb (500 g) skinless, boneless chicken thighs, trimmed of fat and halved crosswise
1 yellow (brown) onion, chopped
1¹/₂ tablespoons unsalted butter
¹/₃ cup (1¹/₂ oz/45 g) desiccated coconut
2 tablespoons Coondapour Masala (page 30)
1 teaspoon salt
¹/₂ cup (4 fl oz/125 ml) coconut milk
Juice of 1 lemon

For Tempering
1¹/₂ tablespoons unsalted butter
1 tablespoon vegetable oil
1 yellow (brown) onion, chopped
1 tablespoon minced garlic

This recipe is a specialty of the Usha restaurant in Mangalore, which is also famous for its kori gasi (page 68). I learned to make this recipe while training there, just before the Taj Group opened the Karavalli restaurant in Bangalore.

1. In a heavy-bottomed saucepan, combine chicken, onion, butter, coconut, coondapour masala, salt and coconut milk. Bring to a simmer over medium–low heat, cover and cook until chicken is almost tender, about 15 minutes. Uncover and continue to simmer until sauce is thick and coats chicken, 5–10 minutes. Remove pan from heat and stir in lemon juice. Set aside.
2. To make tempering: In a small frying pan, heat butter and oil over medium–high heat. Add onion and cook, stirring often, until onion starts to caramelize, 5–6 minutes. Stir in garlic and continue to cook for 1 minute longer.
3. Transfer chicken to a serving dish and pour tempering over top. Serve immediately.

Serves 4 as starter
Serves 6–8 as starter with 1 other starter
Serves 8–10 as starter with all 3 starters

Chicken with coconut (front),
lamb with green masala (back)

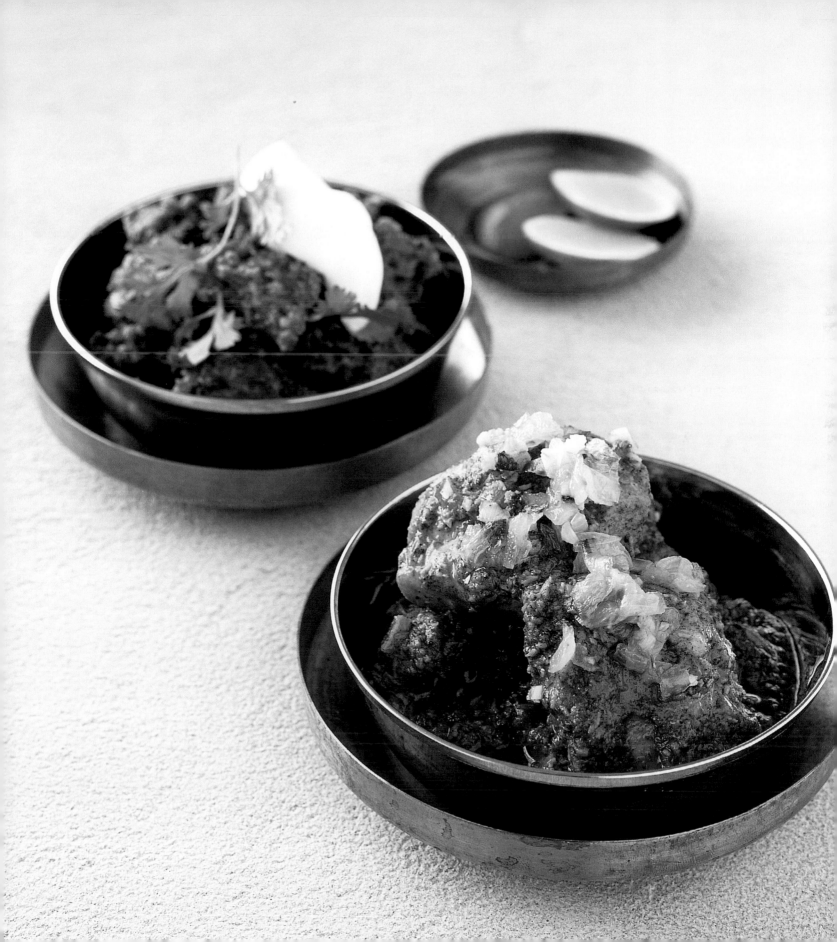

Lamb with green masala
Massa hasiru

For Green Masala
1 bunch fresh cilantro (fresh coriander), leaves, stems and roots roughly chopped
1 yellow (brown) onion, chopped
10 fresh mild long green chilies, roughly chopped
1-inch (2.5-cm) piece fresh ginger, peeled and roughly chopped
4 cloves garlic
2-inch (5-cm) piece cinnamon stick
2 green cardamom pods
1 teaspoon coriander seeds
1/2 teaspoon ground turmeric

1/4 cup (2 oz/60 g) unsalted butter
1 yellow (brown) onion, finely chopped
1 teaspoon salt
1 lb (500 g) boneless lamb shoulder (blade), cut into 1-inch (2.5-cm) cubes
1/4 cup (2 fl oz/60 ml) vegetable stock
Juice of 1 lime
Plain whole-milk yogurt, for serving
Lime wedges, for serving

My friend K.K. Shiva calls this his "secret" lamb recipe.

1. To make green masala: In a food processor, combine cilantro, onion, chilies, ginger and garlic. Process until a fine paste forms. In a spice grinder, combine cinnamon, cardamom and coriander and grind to a fine powder. Add to processor along with turmeric. Process until well combined. Set aside.
2. In a heavy-bottomed saucepan, melt butter over medium–low heat. Add onion and salt and cook, stirring occasionally, until onion is softened, 10–15 minutes.
3. Raise heat to high, add lamb and cook, stirring and tossing, until meat is seared, 3–4 minutes. Add stock and bring to a simmer. Reduce heat to medium–low, cover partially and cook until lamb is very tender, 45–60 minutes.
4. Add green masala to lamb and stir well. Cook uncovered, stirring often, for 10 minutes longer to blend flavors. Taste and adjust seasoning with salt.
5. Transfer to a serving dish and drizzle with lime juice. Serve hot, with yogurt and lime wedges.

Serves 4 as starter
Serves 6–8 as starter with 1 other starter
Serves 8–10 as starter with all 3 starters

Dry-fried shellfish
Marvai ajadina

3 tablespoons vegetable oil
1 tablespoon coriander seeds
2 teaspoons cumin seeds
1/2 teaspoon fenugreek seeds
2 dried red chilies
1/2 teaspoon black peppercorns
1/3 cup (1 1/2 oz/45 g) desiccated coconut
1/4 teaspoon ground turmeric
2–3 tablespoons water
1 yellow (brown) onion, chopped
1 teaspoon salt
24 medium shrimp (prawns), peeled and deveined, with tail segments intact if desired
1 teaspoon tamarind concentrate
Juice of 1/2 lemon

For Tempering
2 tablespoons vegetable oil
1 yellow (brown) onion, chopped
1 tablespoon minced garlic

Mixed salad greens for serving

I learned to make this dish, an absolute delicacy, in Karvar. Try making it with crab in place of the shrimp.

1. In a small frying pan, heat 1 tablespoon oil over medium heat. Add coriander, cumin, fenugreek, chilies and peppercorns and cook, stirring, until fragrant, 2–3 minutes. Transfer to a plate to cool. Add coconut and turmeric to dry pan and cook, stirring, until coconut is toasted, 1–2 minutes. Set aside on plate to cool.
2. Place toasted whole spices in a spice grinder and grind to a powder. Transfer ground spices to a small food processor. Add coconut and turmeric to processor and process to combine. Add 2 tablespoons water and process to form a smooth paste, adding more water as needed. Set spice paste aside.
3. In a medium frying pan, heat remaining 2 tablespoons oil over medium–low heat. Add onion and salt and cook uncovered, stirring occasionally, until onion is softened, 10–15 minutes.
4. Raise heat to high, add spice paste and cook, stirring, for 2 minutes. Add shrimp and cook, stirring and tossing, just until cooked through, 4–5 minutes.
5. In a small bowl, stir together tamarind and lemon juice, and then stir into shrimp mixture. Remove from heat and cover to keep hot.
6. To make tempering: In a small frying pan, heat oil over medium–high heat. Add onion and cook, stirring often, until onion starts to caramelize, 5–6 minutes. Stir in garlic and cook for 1 minute longer.
7. Transfer hot shrimp mixture to serving dish and pour tempering over top. Serve immediately, with salad greens alongside.

Serves 4 as starter
Serves 6–8 as starter with 1 other starter
Serves 8–10 as starter with all 3 starters

Main Dishes

Chicken biryani

1 cup (8 fl oz/250 ml) vegetable oil
4 yellow (brown) onions, halved and thinly sliced
1 teaspoon salt, plus extra for cooking rice
2¼ cups (1 lb/500 g) basmati rice
4 fresh mild long green chilies, slit lengthwise
1½ tablespoons grated fresh ginger
1½ tablespoons minced garlic
1 cup (8 oz/250 g) plain whole-milk yogurt, whisked until smooth
1 whole chicken, 3 lb (1.5 kg), cut into 10 pieces, or 2 lb (1 kg) chicken pieces
¼ cup (1 oz/30 g) unsalted roasted cashew nuts, chopped
¼ cup (1½ oz/45 g) raisins, chopped
Juice of 1 lemon
Leaves from 1 bunch fresh cilantro (fresh coriander), chopped
Leaves from 1 small bunch fresh mint, chopped
2 teaspoons Nilgiri's Garam Masala (page 28)
1 teaspoon saffron threads, soaked in 1½ tablespoons hot milk for 10 minutes

Sweet Mango Pickle (page 84) and/or Tomato Salad (page 84) for serving

This is my wife Meera's favorite, but she insists that it always be perfect!

1. In a large, heavy-bottomed ovenproof pan, heat oil over medium–low heat. Add onions and 1 teaspoon salt and cook uncovered, stirring occasionally, until onions are dark golden brown, 20–25 minutes. Using a spoon, skim off all excess oil and place in a small bowl.
2. Meanwhile, rinse rice under cold running water until water runs clear. Place in a bowl and cover with plenty of cold water. Set aside for 20 minutes and then drain well. Bring a large saucepan of salted water to a boil, add rice, and cook just until tender, 10–12 minutes. Drain well. Preheat oven to 450°F (230°C/Gas 8).
3. When onions are ready, add chilies, ginger and garlic to pan and continue to cook over medium–low heat, stirring constantly, for 1 minute. Stir in yogurt. Raise heat to high, add chicken and cook, turning occasionally, until chicken changes color on all sides, 4–5 minutes. Add cashew nuts, raisins and lemon juice, reduce heat to low, cover and cook until chicken is about three-fourths cooked, about 15 minutes. Remove pan from heat and stir in cilantro, mint and garam masala.
4. Spoon rice over chicken mixture. Sprinkle with saffron and milk and spoon over reserved oil. Cover rice with a clean, moist kitchen towel or cloth and top with lid. Bake until heated through and flavors are blended, about 10 minutes. Toss through before serving.
5. Serve the biryani hot directly from pan.

Serves 6 with 1 or 2 accompaniments
Serves 6–8 with 1 or 2 accompaniments and 1 vegetarian main dish

Chicken biryani (front), tomato salad (back left), sweet mango pickle (back right)

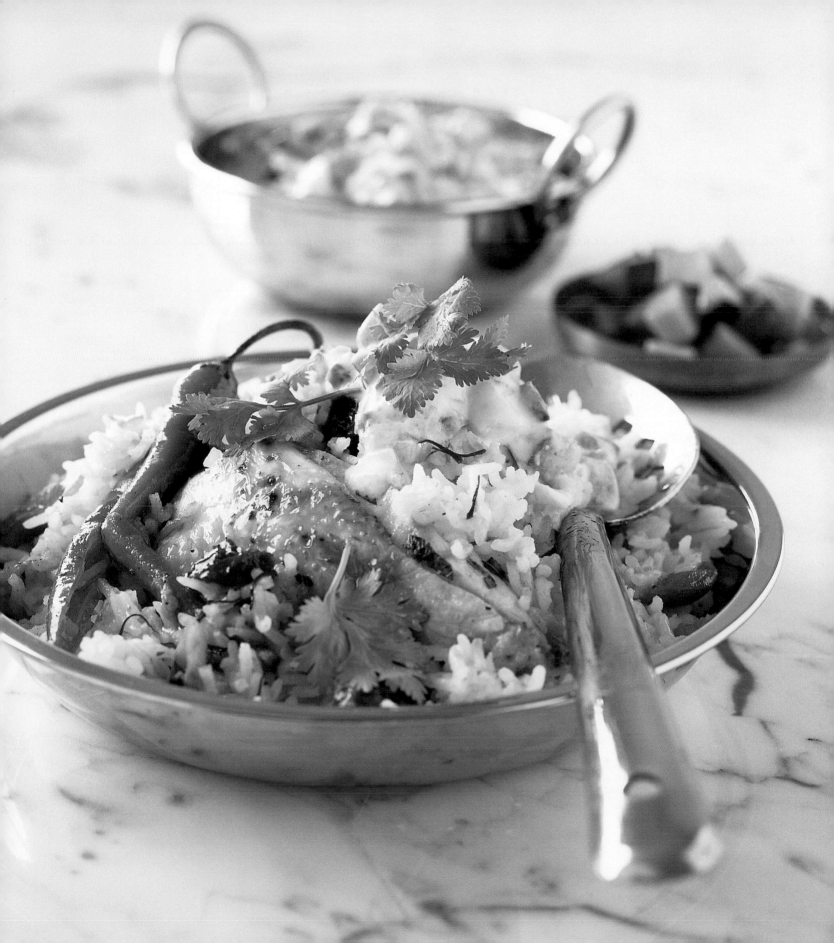

Chicken, Mangalore style
Kori gasi

1 tablespoon vegetable oil
2 tablespoons unsalted butter
2 yellow (brown) onions, chopped
2 teaspoons salt
1 whole chicken, 3 lb (1.5 kg), cut into 10 pieces, or 2 lb (1 kg) chicken pieces
1 can (13 fl oz/400 ml) coconut cream
1 recipe Coondapour Masala (page 30)

For Tempering
1 tablespoon vegetable oil
1 yellow (brown) onion, chopped
1 teaspoon salt
1/2 teaspoon Nilgiri's Garam Masala (page 28)

Juice of 1 lemon

Steamed Basmati Rice (page 141) and/or Rice Pancakes (page 85) for serving
Sweet Mango Pickle (page 84) and/or Tomato Salad (page 84) for serving

This recipe originated at the Usha restaurant in Mangalore and now is the fastest-selling dish at the Karavalli restaurant in Bangalore.

1. In a large, heavy-bottomed saucepan, heat oil and butter over medium–low heat. Add onions and salt and cook uncovered, stirring occasionally, until onions are softened, 10–15 minutes.
2. Raise heat to high, add chicken and cook, turning occasionally, until well browned on all sides, 4–5 minutes. Add coconut cream and coondapour masala and bring to a simmer. Reduce heat to medium and simmer, partially covered, until chicken is tender, about 20 minutes.
3. To make tempering: In a small frying pan, heat oil over medium–high heat. Add onion and salt and cook uncovered, stirring often, until onion is golden brown, 8–10 minutes. Remove from heat and stir in garam masala.
4. Remove saucepan from heat and stir in lemon juice. Transfer to serving dish and pour tempering over top.

Serves 4–6 with rice and/or pancakes, and 1 or 2 accompaniments
Serves 6–8 with rice and/or pancakes, 1 or 2 accompaniments, 1 vegetarian main dish, and 1 meat or seafood main dish

Pepper and garlic chicken
Kozhi milagu

1 cinnamon stick, about 3 inches (7.5 cm) long
2 teaspoons green cardamom pods
1 teaspoon whole cloves
1 teaspoon whole peppercorns
1/3 cup (1/2 oz/15 g) chopped fresh cilantro (fresh coriander)
36 fresh curry leaves
Juice of 1 1/2 lemons
1 fresh mild long green chili, finely chopped
2 tablespoons minced garlic
1 tablespoon grated fresh ginger
2 teaspoons tamarind concentrate
1 teaspoon ground turmeric
1 teaspoon salt
2 lb (1 kg) skinless, boneless chicken thighs, trimmed of fat and halved crosswise
2 tablespoons vegetable oil
1/4 cup (2 oz/60 g) unsalted butter

Mixed salad greens for serving
Steamed Basmati Rice (page 141) or Coconut Rice (page 85) and/or Rice Pancakes (page 85) for serving
Sweet Mango Pickle (page 84) and/or Tomato Salad (page 84) for serving

The Nagarjuna restaurant in Bangalore is renowned for this Tamil Nadu dish. This is my version.

1. In a spice grinder, combine cinnamon, cardamom, cloves and peppercorns and grind to a fine powder. Transfer ground spices to a small food processor and add cilantro, curry leaves, juice of 1 lemon, chili, garlic, ginger, tamarind, turmeric and salt. Process until a paste forms.
2. Place chicken pieces in a glass or ceramic bowl. Add remaining juice of 1/2 lemon and turn to coat. Let stand for 5 minutes. Add paste and turn chicken to coat well. Set aside for 15 minutes to marinate.
3. Line a large bamboo steamer basket with parchment (baking) paper. Arrange chicken in a single layer on paper – you may have to cook in 2 batches. Place basket over a wok or other pan of barely simmering water. Cover and steam until chicken is cooked through and tender, 12–15 minutes. Transfer chicken to a plate. Repeat if cooking in 2 batches.
4. In a large frying pan, heat oil and butter over medium–high heat. Add chicken and cook, turning once, until golden brown on both sides, 1–2 minutes on each side. Serve hot with salad greens alongside.

Serves 4–6 with rice and/or pancakes, salad, and 1 or 2 accompaniments
Serves 6–8 with rice and/or pancakes, salad, 1 or 2 accompaniments, and Coconut and Mustard Lentils (page 81) and 1 seafood or meat main dish

Fennel and chili lamb
Erachi porichathu

2 lb (1 kg) boneless lamb shoulder (blade), cut into 1-inch (2.5-cm) cubes
1¹/₂ tablespoons aniseed
1¹/₂ tablespoons fennel seeds
1 tablespoon chili powder
1 tablespoon ground turmeric
3 teaspoons minced garlic
1 teaspoon salt
2 tablespoons vegetable oil

Steamed Basmati Rice (page 141) or Coconut Rice (page 85) and/or Rice Pancakes (page 85) for serving
Sweet Mango Pickle (page 84) and/or Tomato Salad (page 84) for serving

This dish is best when accompanied with coconut-scented rice.

1. In a large bowl, combine lamb, aniseed, fennel, chili powder, turmeric, garlic and salt and stir well to coat lamb evenly. Cover and set aside for 15 minutes to marinate.
2. Preheat oven to 300°F (150°C/Gas 2). In a large, wide, heavy-bottomed ovenproof saucepan, heat 1 tablespoon oil over high heat. Add half of marinated meat and cook, stirring and tossing, until meat is well browned, 3–4 minutes. Transfer to a bowl. Repeat with remaining 1 tablespoon oil and meat. Return all meat to pan.
3. Cover pan and bake, stirring occasionally, until meat is very tender, 60–70 minutes. Remove from oven, taste and adjust with salt if necessary, and then re-cover and set aside for 10 minutes to rest before serving.

Serves 4–6 with rice and/or pancakes, 1 or 2 accompaniments, and 1 vegetarian main dish
Serves 6–8 with rice and/or pancakes, 1 or 2 accompaniments, 1 vegetarian main dish, and 1 chicken or seafood main dish

Ginger lamb curry
Inji kari kozhambu

2 lb (1 kg) lamb cut from leg, cut into 1-inch (2.5-cm) pieces
2 tablespoons plus 2 teaspoons grated fresh ginger
2 teaspoons coriander seeds, ground in spice grinder
1/2–1 teaspoon chili powder
1 teaspoon ground turmeric
2 tablespoons vegetable oil
3 yellow (brown) onions, chopped
1 teaspoon salt
2-inch (5-cm) piece cinnamon stick
3 whole cloves
4 green cardamom pods
2 teaspoons crushed garlic
4 fresh mild long green chilies, slit lengthwise
1 can (13 fl oz/400 ml) coconut milk
Juice of 1 lemon
Leaves from 1 bunch fresh cilantro (fresh coriander), chopped

Steamed Basmati Rice (page 141) and/or Rice Pancakes (page 85) for serving
Sweet Mango Pickle (page 84) and/or Tomato Salad (page 84) for serving

I first had a taste of this dish in my friend Illango's house in Madras and still can't get it out of my head.

1. In a large bowl, combine lamb, 2 tablespoons ginger, coriander, chili powder and turmeric. Stir well to combine. Set aside for 1 hour to marinate.
2. In a large, heavy-based saucepan, heat oil over medium–low heat. Add onions and salt and cook uncovered, stirring occasionally, until onions are softened, 10–15 minutes. Raise heat to medium, add cinnamon, cloves and cardamom and cook, stirring, until fragrant, 2–3 minutes. Add garlic, remaining 2 teaspoons ginger and chilies and cook, stirring, for 1 minute.
3. Raise heat to high, add lamb and cook, turning occasionally, until well browned, 3–4 minutes. Add coconut milk and bring to a simmer. Reduce heat to low, cover partially and cook, stirring occasionally, until lamb is very tender, about 1 1/2 hours.
4. Remove pan from heat and stir in lemon juice. Taste and adjust seasoning with salt if necessary. Transfer to serving dish and top with cilantro. Serve hot.

Serves 4–6 with rice and/or pancakes, 1 or 2 accompaniments, and Coconut and Mustard Lentils (page 81)
Serves 6–8 with rice and/or pancakes, 1 or 2 accompaniments, Coconut and Mustard Lentils (page 81) or 1 vegetarian main dish, and 1 chicken or seafood main dish

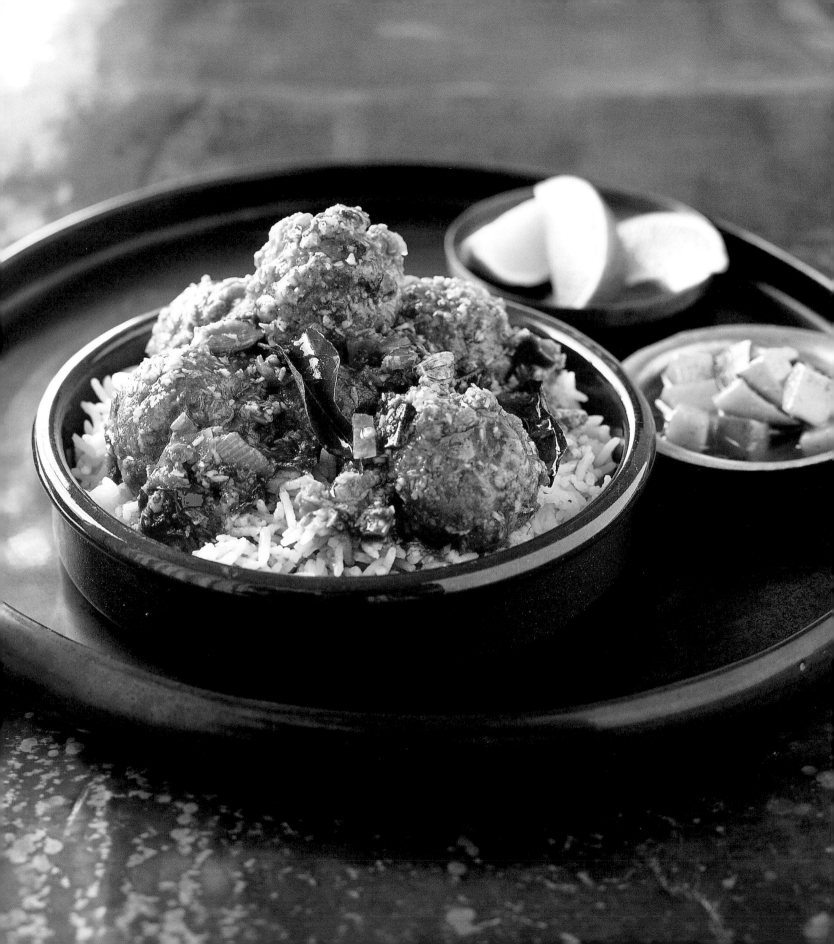

Meatball curry
Kyma urundai kari kozhambu

For Meatballs
1 teaspoon coriander seeds
2 whole cloves
2 inch (5 cm) piece cinnamon stick
1 lb (500 g) ground (minced) lamb
1 teaspoon grated fresh ginger
1 teaspoon minced garlic
1/2 teaspoon ground turmeric
1/2 teaspoon chili powder
1/4 cup (11/2 oz/45 g) fine semolina
1 egg, lightly whisked
1 teaspoon salt

For Sauce
2 tablespoons vegetable oil
2 yellow (brown) onions, finely chopped
1 teaspoon salt
10 fresh curry leaves
2 whole cloves
2-inch (5-cm) piece cinnamon stick
2 green cardamom pods
11/2 teaspoons chili powder
2 teaspoons coriander seeds, ground
in spice grinder
1 tablespoon grated fresh ginger
1 tablespoon minced garlic
4 large, ripe tomatoes, chopped
1/2 cup (2 oz/60 g) desiccated coconut
2 teaspoons cumin seeds, ground
in spice grinder
11/2 cups (12 fl oz/375 ml) vegetable
stock
Juice of 1/2 lime

Leaves from 1 bunch fresh cilantro
(fresh coriander), chopped (optional)

Steamed Basmati Rice (page 141)
and/or Rice Pancakes (page 85)
for serving
Sweet Mango Pickle (page 85) and/or
Tomato Salad (page 84) for serving

1. To make meatballs: In a spice grinder, combine coriander, cloves and cinnamon and grind to a fine powder. In a bowl, combine lamb, ground spices, ginger, garlic, turmeric, chili powder, semolina, egg, and salt. Mix until well combined. Shape tablespoonfuls of mixture into balls. Set aside.
2. To make sauce: In a large, heavy-bottomed frying pan, heat oil over medium–low heat. Add onions and salt and cook uncovered, stirring occasionally, until onions are softened, 10–15 minutes. Add curry leaves, cloves, cinnamon and cardamom and cook, stirring, until fragrant, 2–3 minutes. Stir in chili powder, coriander, ginger and garlic and cook, stirring, for 1 minute. Remove from heat.
3. In a small food processor, combine tomatoes, coconut and cumin and process until well combined. Add to pan holding onion mixture and add stock. Taste and adjust seasoning with salt if necessary. Place over medium heat and simmer, uncovered, for 10 minutes to thicken slightly and blend flavors.
4. Carefully add meatballs to sauce, cover and cook over low heat until meatballs are tender, about 15 minutes.
5. Remove pan from heat and stir in lime juice. Transfer to serving dish and top with cilantro. Serve hot.

Serves 4–6 with rice and/or pancakes and 1 or 2 accompaniments
Serves 6–8 with rice and/or pancakes, 1 or 2 accompaniments, 1 vegetarian main dish, and 1 chicken or meat main dish

Meatball curry served with steamed basmati rice, sweet mango pickle and lime wedges

Fish in tamarind and coondapour masala
Kane gasi

2 tablespoons vegetable oil
1 yellow (brown) onion, finely chopped
1 teaspoon salt
1 recipe Coondapour Masala (page 30)
1 can (13 fl oz/400 ml) coconut cream
1 teaspoon tamarind concentrate
1¹/₂ lb (750 g) white fish fillets
such as snapper or cod, cut into
1-inch (2.5-cm) pieces

Steamed Basmati Rice (page 141)
and/or Rice Pancakes (page 85)
for serving
Sweet Mango Pickle (page 84) and/or
Tomato Salad (page 84) for serving

In Mangalore, this traditional dish is made with ladyfish, but here I have used white fish fillets because of their greater availability.

1. In a large frying pan, heat oil over medium–low heat. Add onion and salt and cook uncovered, stirring often, until onion is softened, 10–15 minutes.
2. Add coondapour masala and coconut cream, raise heat to medium and bring to a simmer. Stir in tamarind and then add fish. Cook until fish is just cooked and flakes when tested with a fork, 7–8 minutes.
3. Taste and adjust seasoning with salt. Transfer to a serving dish and serve hot.

Serves 4–6 with rice and/or pancakes and 1 or 2 accompaniments
Serves 6–8 with rice and/or pancakes, 1 or 2 accompaniments, 1 vegetarian main dish, and 1 chicken or meat main dish

Fish in mustard-and-tamarind tomato sauce
Meen mulakittathu

3 tablespoons vegetable oil
¹/₂ teaspoon fenugreek seeds
¹/₂ teaspoon black or brown
mustard seeds
5 yellow (brown) onions, halved
and thinly sliced
20 fresh curry leaves
1 teaspoon salt
2 fresh mild long green chilies,
slit lengthwise
1¹/₂ tablespoons minced garlic
1 large, ripe tomato, about
7 oz (220 g), roughly chopped
1–2 teaspoons chili powder
¹/₂ teaspoon ground turmeric
³/₄ cup (6 fl oz/180 ml) fish stock
or water
1 teaspoon tamarind concentrate
1¹/₂ lb (750 g) white fish fillets
such as snapper or cod, cut into
serving-sized portions if large

Steamed Basmati Rice (page 141) or
Coconut Rice (page 85) and/or Rice
Pancakes (page 85) for serving
Sweet Mango Pickle (page 84) and/or
Tomato Salad (page 84) for serving

You will find this dish on the tables of the Muslim community of Kerala. It is best eaten the day after it is made.

1. In a heavy-bottomed saucepan, heat oil over medium heat. Add fenugreek and mustard seeds and cook, stirring, until seeds pop, 1–2 minutes.
2. Add onions, curry leaves and salt and cook uncovered, stirring occasionally, until onions are softened, 10–15 minutes. Add chilies and garlic and cook, stirring, for 1 minute. Add tomato, chili powder (use larger amount if you want more heat) and turmeric and cook, stirring, until tomato breaks down and oil separates, 5–6 minutes.
3. Add stock or water and bring to a simmer. Stir in tamarind concentrate. Add fish fillets and cook over medium heat until fish is just cooked and flakes when tested with a fork, 7–8 minutes.
4. Transfer to a serving dish and serve hot.

Serves 4–6 with rice and/or pancakes and 1 or 2 accompaniments
Serves 6–8 with rice and/or pancakes, 1 or 2 accompaniments, Stuffed Eggplant (page 80) or Coconut and Mustard Lentils (page 81) and 1 chicken or meat main dish

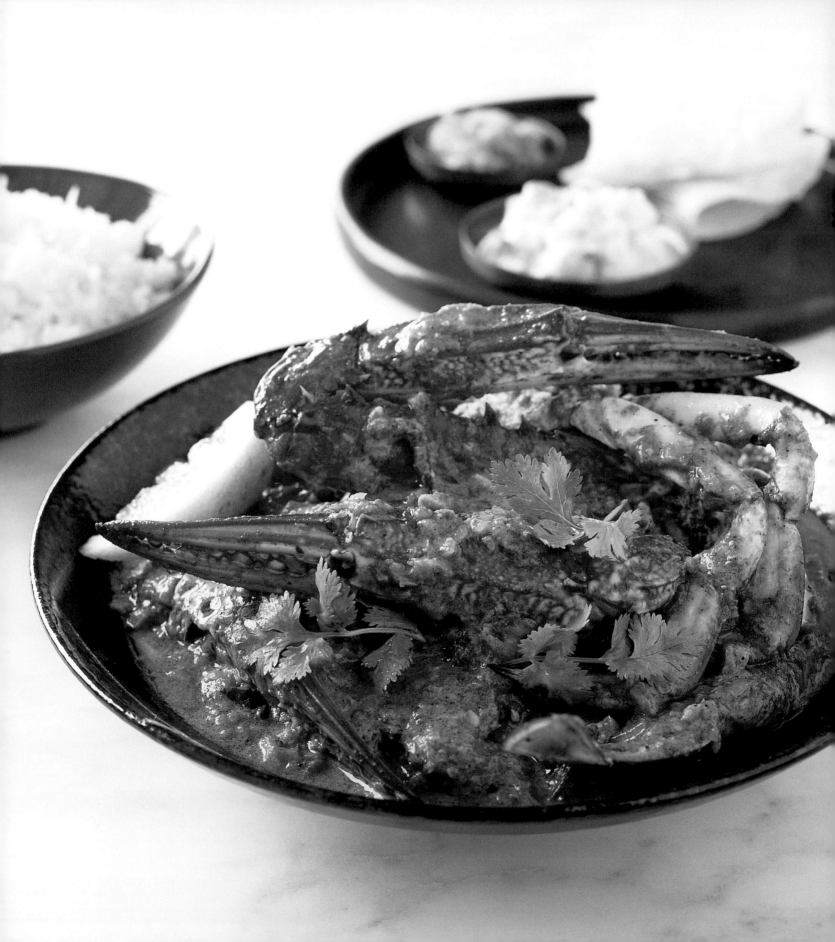

Crab curry
Nandu kari kozhambu

2¹/₂ lb (1.25 kg) soft-shell or blue swimmer crabs (about 4 crabs)
4 tablespoons (2 fl oz/60 ml) vegetable oil
1 large yellow (brown) onion, halved and thinly sliced
4 large, ripe tomatoes, chopped
5 fresh mild long green chilies, slit lengthwise
1-inch (2.5-cm) piece fresh ginger, peeled and sliced
6 cloves garlic
1 teaspoon aniseed
1 teaspoon coriander seeds
6 black peppercorns
1-inch (2.5-cm) piece cinnamon stick
3 green cardamom pods
¹/₂ teaspoon cumin seeds
¹/₄ cup (1 oz/30 g) desiccated coconut
10 fresh curry leaves
1 teaspoon chili powder
¹/₂ teaspoon ground turmeric
1 cup (8 fl oz/250 ml) fish or vegetable stock
¹/₂ cup (4 fl oz/125 ml) coconut cream
1 teaspoon salt
¹/₂ cup (³/₄ oz/20 g) fresh cilantro (fresh coriander) leaves
Lemon wedges for serving

Steamed Basmati Rice (page 141) and/or Rice Pancakes (page 85) for serving
Sweet Mango Pickle (page 84) and/or Tomato Salad (page 84) for serving

Crab curry with steamed basmati rice, sweet mango pickle, tomato salad and rice pancakes

This soft-shell crab dish is yet another favorite of mine.

1. Remove large top shell from each crab. Remove fibrous matter from inside crab and discard. Rinse crabs well. Using a sharp knife, cut each crab into quarters. Use a meat mallet to crack the shells on the legs. This will make meat easier to get out once cooked. Set aside.
2. In a large, shallow, wide pan, heat 2 tablespoons oil over medium–low heat. Add onion, tomatoes, chilies, ginger and garlic and cook, uncovered, stirring often, until onion is softened, 10–15 minutes. Transfer to a plate. Rinse and dry pan and reserve.
3. Heat a nonstick frying pan over medium heat. Add aniseed, coriander, peppercorns, cinnamon, cardamom and cumin and dry-roast, stirring, until fragrant, 2–3 minutes. Transfer to a spice grinder. Add coconut and curry leaves to pan and cook, stirring, until coconut is golden brown, 1–2 minutes. Set aside to cool slightly. Grind spices to a fine powder. Transfer to a food processor and add toasted coconut and curry leaves, onion mixture, chili powder and turmeric. Process until well combined.
4. In reserved pan, heat remaining 2 tablespoons oil over medium-low heat. Add spice mixture and cook, stirring, until fragrant, 2–3 minutes. Pour in stock, add crab, and stir to coat. Cover and cook, turning crab occasionally, until crab becomes vibrant orange-red, about 15 minutes. Remove pan from heat and set aside, covered, for 5 minutes to finish cooking.
5. Transfer crab pieces to a plate. Stir coconut cream and salt into sauce remaining in pan. Taste and adjust seasoning with salt. Return crab to pan and turn to coat pieces with sauce.
6. Serve crab topped with cilantro and lemon wedges.

Serves 4 with rice and/or pancakes and 1 or 2 accompaniments
Serves 6–8 with rice and/or pancakes, 1 or 2 accompaniments, Fried Potatoes with Dill (page 83) or Coconut and Mustard Lentils (page 81) and 1 chicken or meat main dish

Note: A large, deep, wide pan is ideal for this recipe, as the crab pieces form only a thin layer and a wide pan will ensure they cook evenly. If you use a smaller pan, the crab will take longer to cook.

Vegetable stew
Vegetable ishtew

2 tablespoons vegetable oil
1¹/₂ teaspoons black peppercorns
4 whole star anise
2 yellow (brown) onions, halved and
thinly sliced
1 teaspoon salt
6 fresh mild long green chilies,
slit lengthwise
1 teaspoon grated fresh ginger
1 teaspoon minced garlic
8 oz (250 g) potatoes, chopped
8 oz (250 g) ripe tomatoes, chopped
8 oz (250 g) carrots, peeled and
chopped
1 can (13 fl oz/400 ml) coconut cream
8 oz (250 g) green beans, chopped
Leaves from ¹/₂ bunch fresh cilantro
(fresh coriander), chopped

Steamed Basmati Rice (page 141)
and/or Rice Pancakes (page 85)
for serving
Sweet Mango Pickle (page 84) and/or
Tomato Salad (page 84) for serving

1. In a heavy-bottomed saucepan, heat oil over medium heat. Add peppercorns and star anise and cook, stirring, until fragrant, 2–3 minutes. Add onions and salt and cook uncovered, stirring occasionally, until onions are softened, 10–15 minutes.
2. Add chilies, ginger and garlic to pan and cook, stirring, for 1 minute. Add potatoes, tomatoes and carrots. Cook covered over medium heat, stirring occasionally, for about 15 minutes. Add coconut cream and bring to a simmer. Add beans and simmer, uncovered, until vegetables are tender and sauce has thickened, 15 minutes.
3. Transfer to a serving dish and top with cilantro. Serve hot.

Serves 4–6 with rice and/or pancakes, 1 or 2 accompaniments, and Coconut and Mustard Lentils (page 81)
Serves 6–8 (vegetarian menu) with rice and/or pancakes, 1 or 2 accompaniments, Coconut and Mustard Lentils (page 81), and Fried Potatoes with Dill (page 83)
Serves 6–8 (meat menu) with rice and/or pancakes, 1 or 2 accompaniments, Coconut and Mustard Lentils (page 81) or Fried Potatoes with Dill (page 83), and 1 chicken, meat or seafood main dish

Vegetable stew (center),
sweet mango pickle (front right)

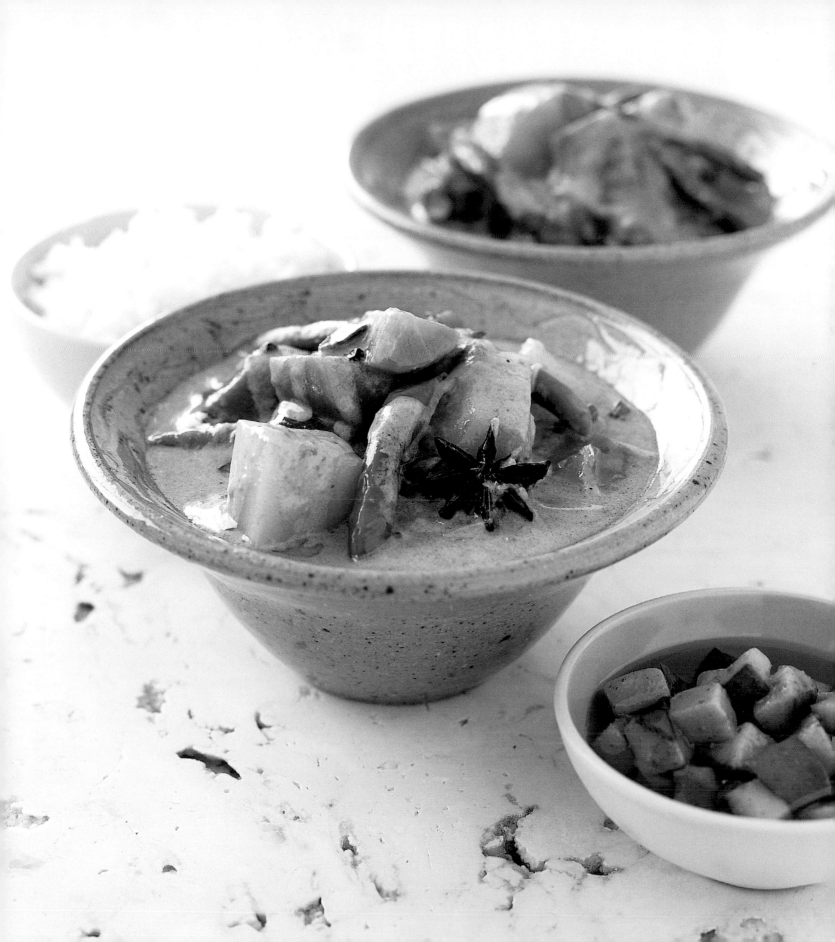

Stuffed eggplant
Kathrikkai varuval

1 lb (500 g) small, round purple eggplants (aubergines)
1 tablespoon plus ¹/₂ cup (4 fl oz/125 ml) vegetable oil
1 large yellow (brown) onion, chopped
1 teaspoon salt
2 teaspoons black peppercorns
1 teaspoon coriander seeds
1 teaspoon cumin seeds
2 dried red chilies
2 whole cloves
2-inch (5-cm) piece cinnamon stick
1 cup (4 oz/125 g) desiccated coconut
2 teaspoons grated fresh ginger
2 teaspoons minced garlic
1 ripe tomato, chopped
1 teaspoon tamarind concentrate
¹/₄ teaspoon ground turmeric
¹/₂ cup (¹/₂ oz/15 g) fresh cilantro (fresh coriander) leaves, chopped

Steamed Basmati Rice (page 141) and/or Rice Pancakes (page 85) for serving
Sweet Mango Pickle (page 84) and/or Tomato Salad (page 84) for serving

1. Starting from blossom (bottom) end of each eggplant, cut a cross, stopping just short of stem. Place in a bowl with water to cover. Set aside.
2. In a large frying pan, heat 1 tablespoon oil over medium–low heat. Add onion and salt and cook uncovered, stirring occasionally, until onion is softened, 10–15 minutes. Transfer to a small food processor.
3. Add peppercorns, coriander, cumin, chilies, cloves and cinnamon to pan over medium heat and cook, stirring, until fragrant, 2–3 minutes. Transfer to a spice grinder. Add coconut to pan and cook, stirring, until golden brown, 1–2 minutes. Remove pan from heat and set aside to cool slightly.
4. Grind spices to a fine powder. Transfer to food processor along with coconut, ginger, garlic, tomato, tamarind and turmeric. Process until a fine paste forms. Preheat oven to 325°F (170°C/Gas 3).
5. Drain eggplant and pat dry with paper towel. Stuff an equal amount of paste into center of each eggplant.
6. In a frying pan, heat ¹/₂ cup (4 fl oz/125 ml) oil over medium heat. When hot, gently lower eggplant into oil. Cook, turning occasionally, until eggplants are browned and start to soften, 5–6 minutes.
7. Transfer eggplants to a baking dish. Pour over hot oil from frying pan. Cover dish with aluminum foil. Bake, turning occasionally, until eggplants are very tender when pierced with a knife tip, 20–30 minutes.
8. Arrange eggplants on platter and top with cilantro. Serve hot.

Serves 4–6 (vegetarian menu) with rice and/or pancakes, 1 or 2 accompaniments, and Coconut and Mustard Lentils (page 81)
Serves 4–6 (meat menu) with rice and/or pancakes, 1 or 2 accompaniments, and 1 chicken, meat or seafood main dish
Serves 6–8 (vegetarian menu) with rice and/or pancakes, 1 or 2 accompaniments, Coconut and Mustard Lentils (page 81) and 1 vegetarian main dish
Serves 6–8 (meat menu) with rice and/or dosa, 1 or 2 accompaniments, Coconut and Mustard Lentils (page 81), and 1 chicken, meat or seafood main dish

Coconut and mustard lentils
Parippu thalichathu

2 cups (14 oz/440 g) split yellow lentils or red lentils
7 cups (56 fl oz/1.75 L) water
1 teaspoon ground turmeric
2 teaspoons vegetable oil
1/2 cup (4 fl oz/125 ml) coconut cream

For Tempering
1 tablespoon vegetable oil
2 teaspoons aniseed
1 teaspoon black or brown mustard seeds
20 fresh curry leaves
1 teaspoon salt
1 teaspoon chili powder
1 1/2 tablespoons minced garlic

Juice of 1/2 lemon
Salt

Steamed Basmati Rice (page 141) and/or Rice Pancakes (page 85) for serving
Sweet Mango Pickle (page 84) and/or Tomato Salad (page 84) for serving

1. Rinse lentils. In a saucepan, combine lentils, water, turmeric and oil. Cover and bring to a boil over high heat. Reduce heat to medium, uncover and simmer, stirring often, until lentils completely break down and all water is absorbed, about 50 minutes. Mixture should be quite thick. Remove from heat and stir in coconut cream. Set aside.

2. To make tempering: In a small frying pan, heat oil over medium heat. Add aniseed and mustard seeds and cook, stirring, until mustard seeds pop, 1–2 minutes. Add curry leaves, salt, chili powder and garlic and cook, stirring, for 1 minute.

3. Pour tempering over dal. Add lemon juice and stir to mix. Taste and adjust seasoning with salt. Transfer to a serving dish and serve hot.

Serves 4–6 (vegetarian menu) with rice and/or pancakes, 1 or 2 accompaniments, and Stuffed Eggplant (page 80)

Serves 4–6 (meat menu) with rice/and or pancakes, 1 or accompaniments, and 1 chicken, meat or seafood main dish

Serves 6–8 (vegetarian menu) with rice, 1 or 2 accompaniments, and 2 vegetarian main dishes

Serves 6–8 (meat menu) with rice, 1 or 2 accompaniments, 1 vegetarian main dish, and 1 chicken, meat or seafood main dish

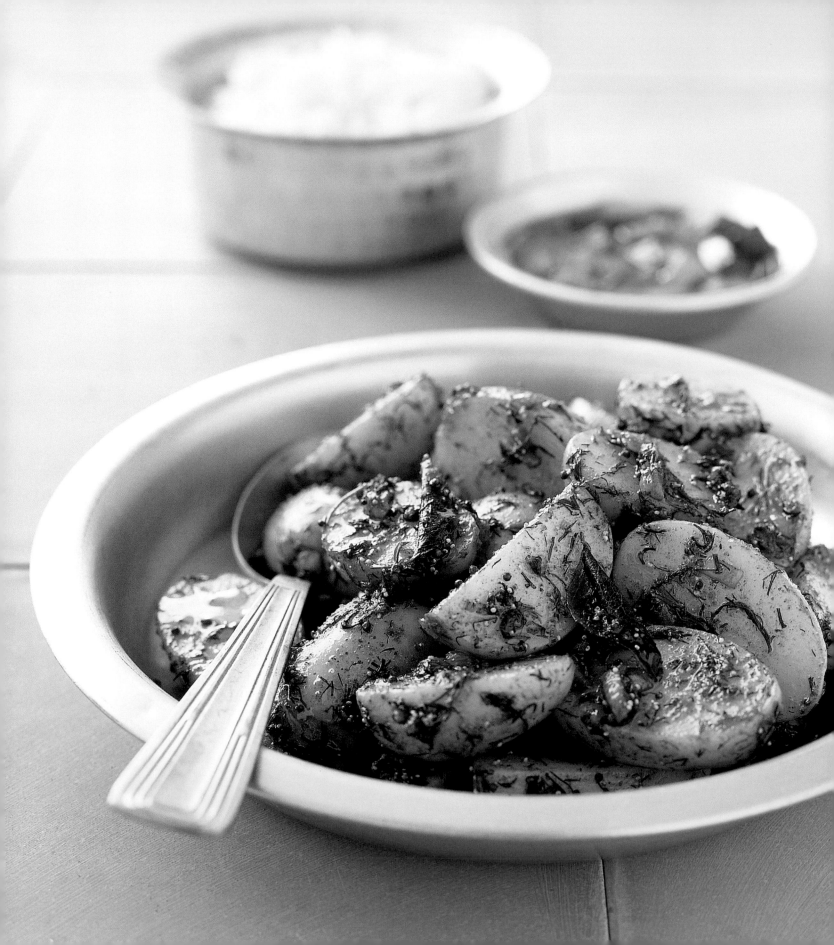

Fried potatoes with dill
Urulakizhangu soyikerrai variyal

1¹/₂ lb (750 g) small potatoes (chats),
unpeeled
¹/₃ cup (3 fl oz/90 ml) vegetable oil
1 teaspoon black or brown
mustard seeds
1 teaspoon split white lentils
(optional)
10 fresh curry leaves
1 yellow (brown) onion, finely chopped
1 tablespoon coriander seeds,
ground in spice grinder
1 teaspoon chili powder
¹/₂ teaspoon ground turmeric
³/₄ cup (1 oz/30 g) finely chopped
fresh dill
1 teaspoon grated fresh ginger
1 teaspoon minced garlic
1 teaspoon salt

Steamed Basmati Rice (page 141) or
Coconut Rice (page 85) for serving
Rice Pancakes (page 85) for serving
(optional)
Sweet Mango Pickle (page 84) and/or
Tomato Salad (page 84) for serving

1. In a saucepan, combine potatoes with plenty of water to cover. Bring to a boil over high heat and boil, uncovered, until just tender, about 10 minutes. Drain and cut into quarters.
2. In a large frying pan, heat oil over medium heat. Add mustard seeds, lentils if using, curry leaves, onion, coriander, chili powder and turmeric and cook, stirring, until onion is lightly golden and spices are fragrant, 4–5 minutes.
3. Add dill, reduce heat to low and cook, stirring, until dill changes color and is fragrant, 3–4 minutes. Add ginger, garlic and salt and cook, stirring, for 1 minute.
4. Add potatoes to pan and cook, stirring and tossing, until potatoes are well coated with spice mix and heated through, 3–4 minutes.
5. Remove pan from heat and taste and adjust seasoning with salt if necessary. Transfer to a serving dish and serve hot.

Serves 4–6 (vegetarian menu) with rice, pancakes (if desired), 1 or 2 accompaniments, and Red Lentil Dal (page 137)
Serves 4–6 (meat menu) with rice, pancakes (if desired), 1 or 2 accompaniments, and 1 chicken, meat or seafood main dish
Serves 6–8 (vegetarian menu) with rice, pancakes (if desired), 1 or 2 accompaniments, Coconut and Mustard Lentils (page 81), and Stuffed Eggplant (page 80)
Serves 6–8 (meat menu) with rice, pancakes (if desired), 1 or 2 accompaniments, Coconut and Mustard Lentils (page 81) or Stuffed Eggplant (page 80), and 1 chicken, meat or seafood main dish

Fried potatoes with dill (front), steamed basmati rice (back left), sweet mango pickle (back right)

Accompaniments

Sweet mango pickle
Methamba

¹/₈ cup (1 oz/30 g) salt
1 teaspoon aniseed
1 teaspoon coriander seeds
¹/₂ teaspoon fenugreek seeds, optional
¹/₂ teaspoon black or brown mustard seeds
Pinch powdered asafetida
1 oz (30 g) jaggery, grated
2 teaspoons chili powder
1 teaspoon ground turmeric
1 lb (500 g) green mangoes, unpeeled, pitted and finely chopped
³/₄–1 cup (6–8 fl oz/180–250 ml) peanut oil, or as needed

A great accompaniment to any meal.

1. In a spice grinder, combine salt, aniseed, coriander, fenugreek and mustard seeds and grind to a fine powder. Transfer to a bowl and stir in asafetida, jaggery, chili powder and turmeric.
2. Add mangoes to spice mix and stir until mango pieces are well coated with spice mix. Stir in oil.
3. Carefully spoon mango mixture into a 4-cup (32-fl oz/1-L) jar with a tight-fitting lid. Carefully pour in oil remaining in bowl, making sure mango mixture is completely covered (if not, pour over a little extra oil). Set aside in a cool, dry place until mango pieces soften, 1–2 weeks.
4. Once opened, refrigerate for up to 6 months, making sure pickle is always completely covered with oil. Use a clean spoon each time you remove pickle to prevent mold from forming.

Makes about 3 cups

Tomato salad
Thakalli pachidi

2 ripe tomatoes, finely chopped
2 yellow (brown) onions, finely chopped
1 fresh mild long green chili, finely chopped
1 tablespoon chopped fresh cilantro (fresh coriander)
¹/₄ teaspoon sugar
Pinch salt
³/₄ cup (6 oz/180 g) plain whole-milk yogurt, whisked until smooth

Another great accompaniment to serve with any meal.

1. In a bowl, combine tomatoes, onions, chili, cilantro, sugar and salt and stir well.
2. Add yogurt and mix until well combined. Serve within 1 hour of making.

Serves 6–8

Coconut rice
Thengai saadam

1 recipe Steamed Basmati Rice (page 141)
2–5 dried red chilies
2 tablespoons coriander seeds
1 teaspoon sesame seeds
1 teaspoon cumin seeds
1 cup (3 oz/90 g) desiccated coconut
1/3 cup (3 fl oz/90 ml) vegetable oil
1 teaspoon black or brown mustard seeds
1 teaspoon split white lentils (optional)
2 tablespoons unsalted roasted peanuts, chopped
15 fresh curry leaves
Juice of 1 lemon
1 teaspoon salt

This rice is delicious with any dish in this chapter that does not contain coconut.

1. Prepare rice as directed and keep hot.
2. Heat a nonstick frying pan over medium heat. Add 1–4 dried chilies (according to taste), coriander, sesame and cumin and dry-roast, stirring often, until fragrant, 3–4 minutes. Set aside to cool slightly. Return pan to medium heat. Add coconut and cook, stirring, until golden brown, 1–2 minutes. Set aside.
3. Add spices to a spice grinder and grind to a fine powder. Set aside.
4. In a large saucepan, heat oil over medium heat. Add mustard seeds and cook, stirring, until seeds pop, 1–2 minutes. Stir in lentils if using, and cook, stirring, until lightly golden, 1–2 minutes. Add 1 chili, peanuts and curry leaves and cook, stirring, until fragrant, about 2 minutes. Stir in lemon juice and salt.
5. Stir ground spices and coconut into mixture in pan and remove from heat. Add rice and toss until well combined. Transfer to a serving dish and serve warm.

Serves 6–8

Variation: To make lemon rice, omit coconut and increase lemon juice to juice of 3 lemons.

Rice pancakes
Neer dosa

2 cups (10 oz/300 g) rice flour
1 teaspoon salt
2 cups (16 fl oz/500 ml) water
Vegetable oil for frying

Serve with any meal as an accompaniment. You can easily double this recipe.

1. In a bowl, stir together rice flour and salt. Stir in enough water to make a very thin batter.
2. Place a frying pan 6 1/2–7 inches (16.5–18 cm) in diameter over high heat and add just enough oil to film bottom of pan, about 1/4 cup (2 fl oz/60 ml). When hot, pour just enough batter into pan to cover bottom with a thin layer and swirl to coat evenly. Cover and cook until just set and lightly golden on bottom, 30–60 seconds. Flip pancake, re-cover and cook until set, about 1 minute longer. Transfer to a plate. Repeat with remaining batter, adding oil to pan and stirring batter before cooking each pancakes. As pancakess are removed from pan, arrange in a single layer. Do not stack, as pancakes are slightly sticky.
3. Serve pancakes warm.

Makes 10

Desserts

Rice pudding with saffron and cardamom
Paal payasam

³/4 cup (5 oz/150 g) long-grain white rice
4 cups (32 fl oz/1 L) whole milk
¹/3 cup (2¹/2 oz/75 g) superfine (caster) sugar
³/4 teaspoon ground green cardamom pods (ground in spice grinder)
¹/4 teaspoon saffron threads, soaked in ¹/4 cup (2 fl oz/60 ml) warm whole milk for 10 minutes
¹/4 cup (1 oz/30 g) slivered blanched almonds

Most southern Indians consider no meal complete without a bowl of this pudding.

1. Rinse rice under cold running water until water runs clear. Place in a bowl and cover with plenty of cold water. Set aside for 20 minutes. Drain well.
2. Meanwhile, in a heavy-bottomed saucepan, heat milk over medium heat, stirring, until milk comes to a boil. Simmer, uncovered, for 15 minutes.
3. Add drained rice and continue to cook until rice is tender, about 20 minutes. Stir in sugar, cardamom and saffron and milk and cook, stirring, until sugar dissolves.
4. Remove from heat and transfer to a single serving bowl or individual bowls. Serve warm topped with almonds.

Serves 4–6

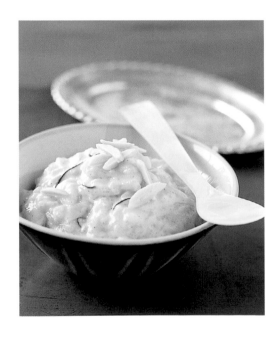

Semolina pudding
Rava kesri

1/3 cup (3 fl oz/90 ml) vegetable oil
2 tablespoons unsalted raw cashew nuts
2 tablespoons raisins
1 cup (6 oz/180 g) fine semolina
2 cups (16 fl oz/500 ml) boiling water
1/2 cup (3 1/2 oz/110 g) superfine (caster) sugar
1/4 teaspoon ground green cardamom pods (ground in spice grinder)
Pinch saffron threads, soaked in 1/4 cup (2 fl oz/60 ml) hot water for 10 minutes

1. In a heavy-bottomed saucepan, heat oil over medium–high heat. When hot, add cashew nuts and raisins and cook, stirring, until golden, 1–2 minutes. Using a slotted spoon, transfer to a plate lined with paper towels.
2. Add semolina to hot oil. Cook, stirring, until semolina turns light golden brown, 5–6 minutes. Remove pan from heat and gradually stir in boiling water.
3. Return pan to medium heat, add sugar, cardamom and saffron and water and stir until well combined and sugar dissolves.
4. Spoon semolina into a 4-cup (32-fl oz/1-L) dish or 1/2-cup (4-fl oz/125-ml) individual dishes. Press down firmly on pudding to pack well, then invert dish or dishes onto individual plates. Cut into serving portions if large dish used. Alternatively, do not unmold. Top servings with raisins and cashew nuts and serve warm or at room temperature.

Serves 6–8

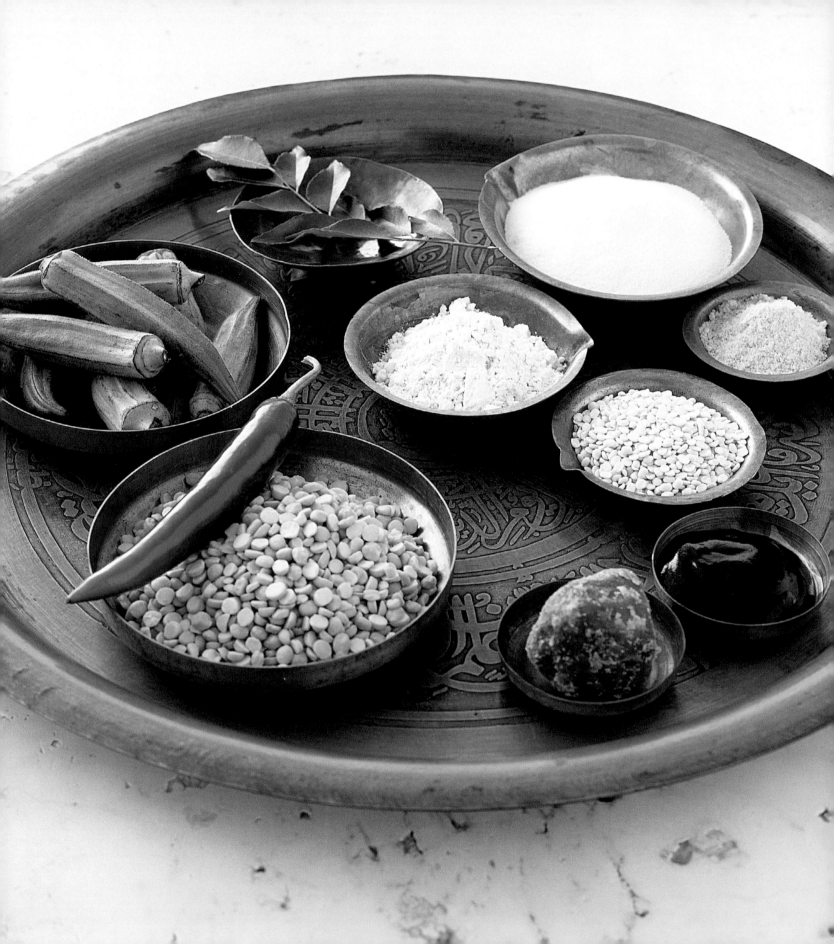

East India

Introduction

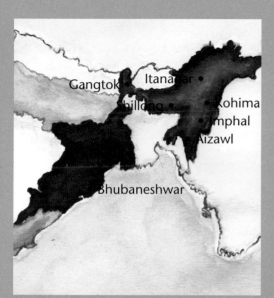

This region, called Poorva Bharath, includes the states of Sikkim, Meghalaya, Arunachal Pradesh, Tripura, Assam and Orissa. It is home to about 300 million people, most of whom have a nomadic way of life except for those living in West Bengal, the north of Andhra Pradesh and Bihar.

Tourism is a booming industry in this region, with visitors being enticed by its spectacular landscape. Overall, the region is quite cold, especially to the far East nearest to the Himalayas. However, the climate ranges from frozen, or tundra conditions, in the north to a tropical climate in the south. Wildlife includes the Himalayan goatlike tahr, the Hoolock gibbon and the almost extinct golden langur (monkey). West Bengal is also the home to the famous Sunbhan tiger.

Visitors are also attracted to Orissa, which is on the east coast of India. This area is often referred to as the Land of Temples, as it boasts up to 1,000 temples in the vicinity. The East Region is also considered the birthplace of Buddhism, and the Dalai Lama is based in this part of the world. Culturally, music plays an important part in the region. In particular, West Bengal is the home of Rabindra music, named after the great Bengali poet, Rabindranath Tagore. From a traditional medicine point of view, some of the most noted Ayurvedic colleges can be found in Orissa.

There is an abundant use of mustard oil, coconut, curry leaf, asafetida and tamarind in the East Region, which are common to this region and distinguish it from the rest of India. Other produce of this region includes figs, bananas, rice, wheat, ginger and pulses. Sikkim, which is situated within the Himalayas, is particularly noted for its cardamom production. Of course, the state of Assam is well known for its teas.

This region is the home of the famous Bengali fish preparation called Maachher Jhole, which is fish cooked in mustard oil with five spices. The cooks of this region have produced a plethora of culinary delights to supplement the simple rice and dal dishes eaten all over India, such as Chickpea Chutney and Fava Beans in Tamarind Sauce.

Although the food from this region is usually chili hot, we have toned down the chilies in the following recipes by changing the flavor from "terribly hot" to "tolerably hot."

Enjoy the heightened flavor of East Indian cooking!

Starters

Curried shrimp
Venchina royyalu

1/3 cup (3 fl oz/90 ml) vegetable oil
3 green cardamom pods
3 whole cloves
1/4 teaspoon aniseed
2 yellow (brown) onions, halved and thinly sliced
1 teaspoon salt
1 1/2 teaspoons coriander seeds, ground in spice grinder
3/4 teaspoon chili powder
3/4 teaspoon ground turmeric
1 1/2 teaspoons grated fresh ginger
1 1/2 teaspoons minced garlic
2 ripe tomatoes, roughly chopped
1/4 cup (2 fl oz/60 ml) water
1 lb (500 g) medium shrimp (prawns), peeled and deveined, tails left intact
2 fresh mild long green chilies, slit lengthwise
Juice of 1 lime
1/4 cup (1/3 oz/10 g) fresh cilantro (fresh coriander) leaves
Lime wedges for serving

This is a version of Tariwale Macchi (page 46) from Andhra Pradesh.

1. In a large frying pan, heat oil over medium heat. Add cardamom, cloves and aniseed and cook, stirring, until fragrant, about 2 minutes.
2. Stir onions and salt into pan, reduce heat to low and cook uncovered, stirring occasionally, until onions are dark golden brown, 20–25 minutes.
3. Add coriander, chili powder and turmeric to pan and cook, stirring, until fragrant, 1–2 minutes. Add ginger and garlic and cook, stirring, for 1 minute. Add tomatoes and water and cook, covered, stirring often, until tomatoes break down, 10–15 minutes.
4. Add shrimp and chilies to pan and simmer until shrimp are just cooked, 2–3 minutes.
5. Remove from heat and stir in lime juice. Transfer to a serving dish and sprinkle with cilantro. Serve hot, with lime wedges.

Serves 4 as a starter
Serves 6–8 as a starter with 1 other starter
Serves 8–10 as a starter with all 3 starters

Curried shrimp (front),
lamb chops with tamarind (back)

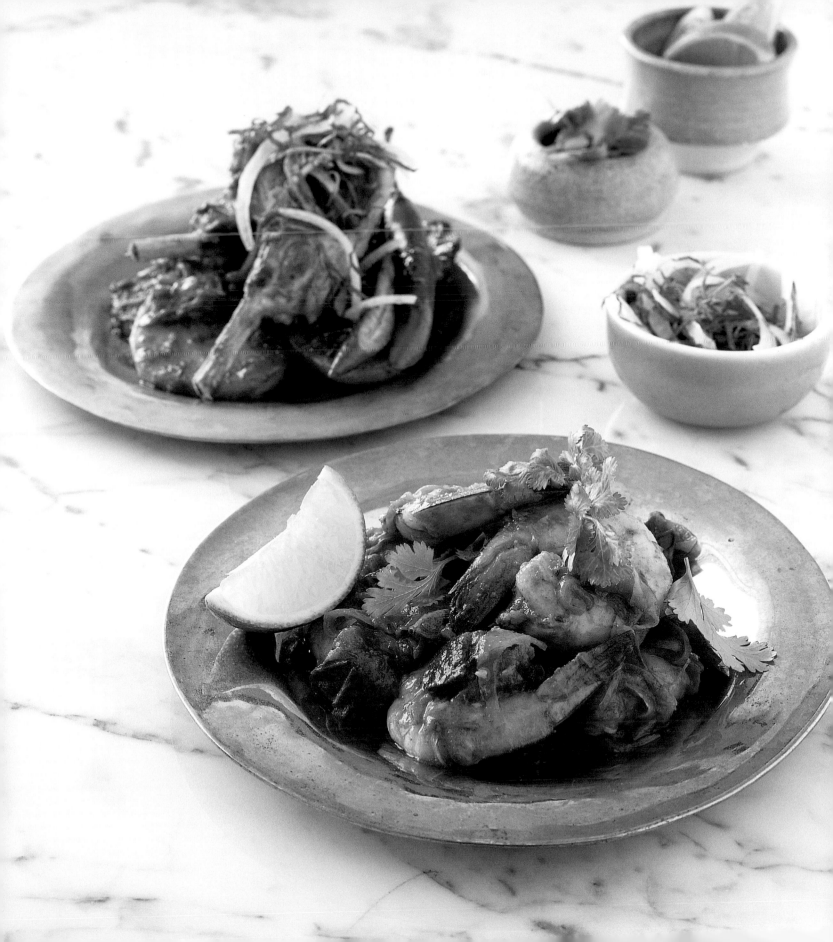

Lamb chops with tamarind
Chintakayi chaap

½ cup (4 fl oz/125 ml) vegetable oil
6 yellow (brown) onions, thinly sliced
1 teaspoon salt
½ teaspoon mustard powder
1 teaspoon grated fresh ginger
3 potatoes, about 4 oz (125 g) each, peeled and cut into slices ¼ inch (6 mm) thick
8 lamb rib chops (cutlets), about 1 lb (500 g) total weight
2 teaspoons tamarind concentrate
1 teaspoon chili powder
3 fresh mild long green chilies, slit lengthwise

For Garnish
1 yellow (brown) onion, halved and thinly sliced
Leaves from ½ bunch fresh mint, finely shredded

Nobody can beat these lamb chops prepared by Vyenkatamma, who uses tamarind, chili and salt to make this recipe special.

1. In a large frying pan, heat oil over medium–low heat. Add onions and salt and cook, uncovered, stirring often, until onions are softened, 10–15 minutes.
2. Raise heat to high and add mustard powder and ginger. Cook, stirring, for 1 minute. Add potatoes and cook, turning often, until lightly golden, about 5 minutes. Add lamb chops and cook, turning once, until browned on both sides, 1–2 minutes on each side.
3. Cover, reduce heat to low and cook until lamb is tender, 5–6 minutes. Transfer lamb to a plate.
4. Add tamarind and chili powder to pan and toss gently to combine with potatoes and other spices. Cover and cook, turning potatoes once, until cooked through and golden brown, 5–10 minutes longer.
5. Return lamb to pan and add chilies. Toss gently until combined.
6. Remove pan from heat and transfer to a serving plate. Garnish with onion and mint and serve hot.

Serves 4 as a starter
Serves 6–8 as a starter with 1 other starter
Serves 8–10 as a starter with all 3 starters

Andhra fish fry
Podichapa

1 lb (500 g) white fish fillets such as snapper or cod, cut into 2-inch (5-cm) pieces
1 teaspoon salt
1 teaspoon ground turmeric
1 teaspoon chili powder
2 teaspoons grated fresh ginger
2 teaspoons minced garlic
1 teaspoon coriander seeds, ground in spice grinder
1 teaspoon cracked black pepper
Juice of 2 limes
Vegetable oil for deep frying
Lemon wedges for serving
Mixed salad greens for serving

Cooks in the coastal areas of Andhra Pradesh prepare this richly spiced fish dish.

1. In a bowl, combine fish, salt and turmeric and toss together until fish is evenly coated. Set aside for 5 minutes.
2. In a small bowl, stir together chili powder, ginger, garlic, coriander, pepper and lime juice.
3. Pour oil to a depth of about 2 inches (5 cm) in a large frying pan and heat over medium heat. When hot, dip fish pieces, a few at a time, into lime juice mixture and carefully slide into hot oil. Cook, turning often, until fish pieces are crisp and cooked through, 2–3 minutes. Using a slotted spoon, transfer to paper towels to drain. Repeat until all fish is cooked.
4. Serve fish hot with lemon wedges and salad.

Serves 4 as a starter
Serves 6–8 as a starter with 1 other starter
Serves 8–10 as a starter with all 3 starters

Main Dishes

Chicken with curry leaves
Kodi gasi

For Masala
4 dried red chilies
1¹/₂ tablespoons coriander seeds
1¹/₂ teaspoons cumin seeds
¹/₂ teaspoon fenugreek seeds
4 black peppercorns
1 cup (4 oz/125 g) desiccated coconut
1 teaspoon minced garlic

1 teaspoon ground turmeric
1 cup (8 fl oz/250 ml) vegetable oil
3 yellow (brown) onions, halved and thinly sliced
40 fresh curry leaves
1 whole chicken, 3 lb (1.5 kg), cut into 10 pieces, or 2 lb (1 kg) chicken pieces
³/₄ cup (6 fl oz/180 ml) water
1 teaspoon salt

Steamed Basmati Rice (page 141) for serving
Chickpea Chutney (page 112), Fava Beans in Tamarind Sauce (page 113), Mango Pickle, Andhra Pradesh Style (page 112) and/or Home-Style Okra Pickle (page 113) for serving

This is the Andhra Pradesh version of the classic chicken dish of Mangalore, Kori Gasi (page 68).

1. To make masala: In a spice grinder, combine chilies, coriander, cumin, fenugreek and peppercorns and grind to a fine powder. Transfer ground spices to a small food processor. Add coconut, garlic and turmeric to processor and process until well combined. Set aside.
2. In a large saucepan, heat oil over medium–high heat. Add half onions and 20 curry leaves and cook, stirring often, until onions and curry leaves are crisp, 8–10 minutes. Using a slotted spoon, transfer to a plate lined with paper towels and set aside.
3. Add remaining onions and 20 curry leaves to pan and cook over medium–high heat, stirring often, until onions are softened, 5–6 minutes. Raise heat to high, add masala and cook, stirring, until fragrant, 1–2 minutes. Add chicken pieces and cook, turning once, until browned, about 2 minutes on each side.
4. Reduce heat to medium–low and stir in water and salt. Cover and cook until chicken is cooked through and tender, about 20 minutes.
5. Taste and adjust seasoning with salt. Transfer chicken to a serving dish and top with fried onions and curry leaves. Serve hot.

Serves 4–6 with rice and 1 or more accompaniments
Serves 6–8 with rice, 1 or more accompaniments, 1 vegetarian main dish, and 1 lamb or seafood main dish

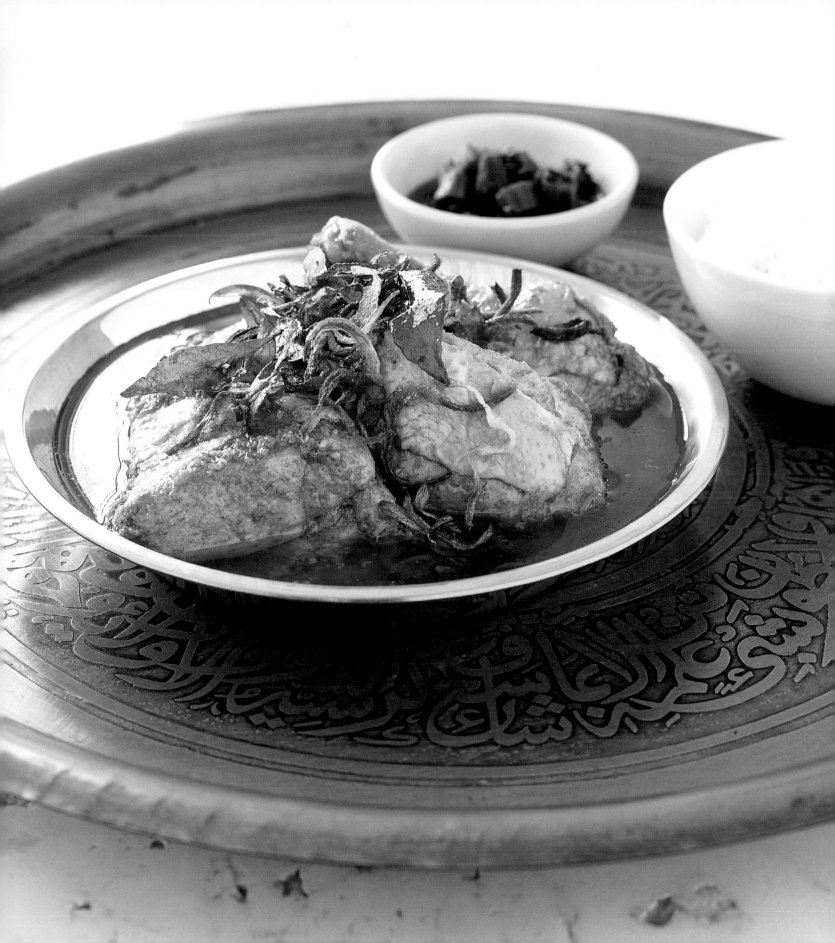

Chicken with tomatoes
Kodi tamatar

¼ cup (2 oz/60 g) unsalted butter
¼ cup (2 fl oz/60 ml) vegetable oil
4 yellow (brown) onions, halved and thinly sliced
1 teaspoon salt
6 brown cardamom pods
1-inch (2.5-cm) piece cinnamon stick
4 whole cloves
1 teaspoon grated fresh ginger
1 teaspoon minced garlic
1 tablespoon chili powder
1 teaspoon coriander seeds, ground in spice grinder
½ teaspoon cumin seeds, ground in spice grinder
¼ teaspoon ground turmeric
2 lb (1 kg) skinless, boneless chicken thighs, trimmed of fat and cut into 1-inch (2.5-cm) pieces
1 lb (500 g) ripe tomatoes, chopped
1 teaspoon tamarind concentrate
60 fresh curry leaves
4 fresh mild long green chilies, slit lengthwise

Steamed Basmati Rice (page 141) for serving
Chickpea Chutney (page 112), Fava Beans in Tamarind Sauce (page 113), Mango Pickle, Andhra Pradesh Style (page 112), and/or Home-Style Okra Pickle (page 113) for serving

In this dish, a favorite of cooks in Andhra Pradesh, tomatoes and tamarind combine to create a delicious result.

1. In a large, heavy-bottomed saucepan, heat butter and oil over medium–low heat. Add onions and salt and cook uncovered, stirring occasionally, until onions are dark golden brown, 20–25 minutes.
2. Add cardamom, cinnamon and cloves and cook, stirring, until fragrant, 2–3 minutes. Add ginger and garlic and cook, stirring, for 1 minute. Add chili powder, coriander, cumin and turmeric and cook, stirring, until aromatic, 2–3 minutes.
3. Raise heat to high, add chicken to pan and cook, stirring, until well browned, 3–4 minutes. Stir in tomatoes and tamarind, reduce heat to low, cover and cook until chicken is cooked through and tender, 15–20 minutes.
4. Stir in curry leaves and chilies, cover and cook over medium heat for 2 minutes. Taste and adjust seasoning with salt if necessary. Transfer to a serving dish and serve hot.

Serves 4–6 with rice and 1 or more accompaniments
Serves 6–8 with rice, 1 or more accompaniments, 1 vegetarian main dish, and 1 lamb or seafood main dish

Chicken in coconut sauce
Kobari kodi pulusu

For Masala
8–10 dried red chilies, broken into small pieces
1/2 cup (2 oz/60 g) desiccated coconut
5 green cardamom pods
1 cinnamon stick, 4 inches (10 cm) long
4 whole cloves
1 tablespoon coriander seeds
3 yellow (brown) onions, halved and thinly sliced
2 teaspoons salt
2 teaspoons minced garlic
1 teaspoon grated fresh ginger

1/2 cup (4 oz/125 g) unsalted butter, cubed
1 whole chicken, 3 lb (1.5 kg)
1 can (13 fl oz/400 ml) coconut milk
1/4 cup (1 1/2 oz/45 g) roasted cashew nuts
Fresh mint sprigs

Steamed Basmati Rice (page 141) for serving
Chickpea Chutney (page 112), Fava Beans in Tamarind Sauce (page 113), Mango Pickle, Andhra Pradesh Style (page 112) and/or Home-Style Okra Pickle (page 113) for serving

Here is a favorite home-style dish, rich with coconut and cashew nuts.

1. To make masala: In a spice grinder, combine chilies, coconut, cardamom, cinnamon, cloves and coriander and grind to a fine powder. Transfer spices to a food processor and add onions, 1 teaspoon salt, garlic and ginger. Process until well combined. Preheat oven to 400°F (200°C/Gas 6).
2. Rinse chicken inside and out and pat dry. Use your fingers to loosen skin from flesh on breast. Rub some of masala under skin of chicken. Stuff remaining masala into cavity of chicken. Using kitchen string, truss chicken, securing wings and legs to body.
3. In a wide, heavy-bottomed ovenproof saucepan, melt butter over medium heat. Add chicken and cook, turning often, until chicken is well browned on all sides, 7–8 minutes.
4. Pour coconut milk over chicken and stir in remaining 1 teaspoon salt. Cover, place in oven and bake until chicken is tender and juices run clear when a thigh joint is pierced with tip of a knife, 40–45 minutes.
5. Remove from oven, and remove chicken from pan. Scoop out masala from cavity into a bowl. Cut chicken into 8 portions, arrange on serving platter, and top with cashew nuts and mint. Serve masala and coconut sauce from pan on side.

Serves 4–6 with rice and 1 or more accompaniments
Serves 6–8 with rice, 1 or more accompaniments, 1 vegetarian main dish, and 1 lamb or seafood main dish

Bengali-style lamb with coconut
Phanthar jhole

2 teaspoons coriander seeds
1 tablespoon plus 2 teaspoons
cumin seeds
3 tablespoons mustard oil
2 lb (1 kg) boneless lamb shoulder
(blade), cut into 1-inch (2.5-cm) pieces
1 tablespoon ground turmeric
2 teaspoons salt, or to taste
2 tablespoons grated fresh ginger
2 tablespoon minced garlic
8 fresh mild long green chilies,
slit lengthwise
1 potato, 4 oz (125 g), peeled and
chopped
1/3 cup (1 1/2 oz/45 g) desiccated
coconut
1 1/2 cups (12 fl oz/375 ml) water
2 teaspoons sugar
Juice of 1 lemon
1/4 cup (1/3 oz/10 g) chopped fresh
cilantro (fresh coriander)

Steamed Basmati Rice (page 141)
for serving
Chickpea Chutney (page 112), Fava
Beans in Tamarind Sauce (page 113),
Mango Pickle, Andhra Pradesh Style
(page 112) and/or Home-Style Okra
Pickle (page 113) for serving

Here, lamb is cooked in mustard oil and simmered with potatoes and coconut for a richly flavored dish.

1. In a spice grinder, combine coriander seeds and 1 tablespoon cumin seeds and grind to a fine powder. Set aside.
2. In a large saucepan, heat oil over high heat. When oil starts to smoke, reduce heat to medium. Add remaining 2 teaspoons whole cumin seeds and cook, stirring, until they start to pop, 1–2 minutes. Raise heat to high and, working in batches, add lamb and cook, stirring and tossing, until well browned,
3–4 minutes. As each batch is ready, transfer to a plate.
3. Return lamb to pan, add turmeric, salt and ground coriander and cumin and cook over high heat, stirring, until fragrant, 1–2 minutes. Add ginger, garlic and chilies, reduce heat to medium and cook, stirring, for 1 minute. Add potatoes, coconut and water, reduce heat to low, cover and simmer until lamb is tender, 45–60 minutes.
4. Remove pan from heat and stir in sugar and lemon juice. Transfer to a serving dish and sprinkle with cilantro. Serve hot.

Serves 4–6 with rice and 1 or more accompaniments
Serves 6–8 with rice, 1 or more accompaniments, 1 vegetarian main dish, and 1 chicken or seafood main dish

Bengali-style lamb with coconut (front),
chickpea chutney (back left),
mango pickle, Andhra Pradesh style (back center),
fava beans in tamarind sauce (back right)

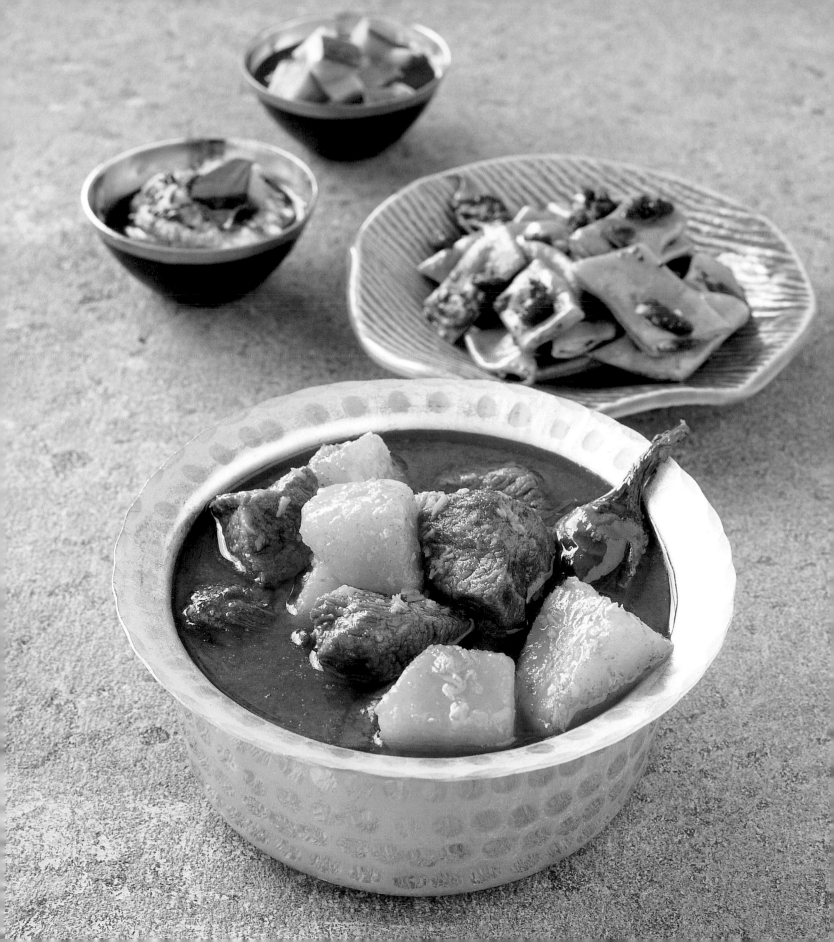

Spiced fried lamb
Podi mamsumu

1 tablespoon coriander seeds
1¹/₂ teaspoons black peppercorns
1¹/₂ cups (12 oz/375 g) plain whole-milk yogurt, whisked until smooth
1 tablespoon chili powder
2 teaspoons Nilgiri's Garam Masala (page 28)
2 teaspoons grated fresh ginger
¹/₂ teaspoon ground turmeric
2 lb (1 kg) boneless lamb shoulder (blade), cut into 1-inch (2.5-cm) pieces
¹/₄ cup (2 oz/60 g) unsalted butter
¹/₄ cup (2 fl oz/60 ml) vegetable oil
3 yellow (brown) onions, halved and thinly sliced
1 teaspoon salt

Steamed Basmati Rice (page 141) or Coconut Rice (page 85) for serving
Chickpea Chutney (page 112), Fava Beans in Tamarind Sauce (page 113), Mango Pickle, Andhra Pradesh Style (page 112) and/or Home-Style Okra Pickle (page 113) for serving

The popular Nilgiri's Kitchen, in Crows Nest, Sydney, is the origin of this spicy lamb and yogurt dish.

1. Heat a nonstick frying pan over medium heat. Add coriander seeds and dry-roast until fragrant, 2–3 minutes. Let cool slightly, then transfer to a spice grinder and grind to a fine powder. Transfer to a bowl. Add peppercorns to spice grinder and grind to a fine powder. Set aside in a separate bowl.
2. Preheat oven to 400°F (200°C/Gas 6). In a bowl, combine ground coriander, yogurt, chili powder, garam masala, ginger and turmeric and stir well to combine. Add lamb and stir well to coat lamb evenly. Set aside for 15 minutes to marinate.
3. In a heavy-bottomed ovenproof saucepan, heat butter and oil over medium–low heat. Add onions and salt and cook uncovered, stirring occasionally, until onions are softened, 10–15 minutes. Add ground pepper and cook, stirring, for 1 minute.
4. Raise heat to high, add lamb and cook, stirring and tossing, until meat is well browned, 3–4 minutes. Cover, place in oven and cook until lamb is very tender, 45–60 minutes.
5. Transfer to a serving dish and serve hot.

Serves 4–6 with rice and 1 or more accompaniments
Serves 6–8 with rice, 1 or more accompaniments, 1 vegetarian main dish, and 1 chicken or seafood main dish

Home-style lamb, liver and kidney
Dumpudu mamsumu

1 cup (8 oz/250 g) plain whole-milk
yogurt, whisked until smooth
$^1/_2$ teaspoon grated fresh ginger
1 teaspoon minced garlic
2 yellow (brown) onions, halved and
thinly sliced
1 teaspoon ground turmeric
1 teaspoon salt
12 oz (375 g) lamb kidneys, trimmed
and cut into 1$^1/_2$-inch (4-cm) pieces
5 oz (150 g) lamb livers, trimmed and
cut into 1$^1/_2$-inch (4-cm) pieces
$^1/_2$ cup (4 fl oz/125 ml) vegetable
stock or water
1$^1/_2$ tablespoons desiccated coconut
$^1/_2$ teaspoon coriander seeds
$^1/_4$ cup (2 fl oz/60 ml) vegetable oil
$^1/_4$ cup (2 oz/60 g) unsalted butter
1-inch (2.5-cm) piece cinnamon stick
2 whole cloves
Leaves from 1 bunch fresh cilantro
(fresh coriander), chopped
$^1/_2$ teaspoon Nilgiri's Garam Masala
(page 28)

Steamed Basmati Rice (page 141)
for serving
Chickpea Chutney (page 112), Fava
Beans in Tamarind Sauce (page 113),
Mango Pickle, Andhra Pradesh Style
(page 112) and/or Home-Style Okra
Pickle (page 113) for serving

On Sunday mornings, I like to eat this dish for breakfast with leftover bread.

1. In a bowl, stir together yogurt, ginger, garlic, onions, turmeric and salt. Add kidneys and livers and stir to coat evenly. Set aside for 10 minutes to marinate.
2. Transfer kidney and liver mixture to a heavy-bottomed saucepan and add stock or water. Place over low heat and cook, uncovered, until all liquid has evaporated and meat is cooked, 10–15 minutes.
3. Meanwhile, heat a small, nonstick frying pan over medium heat. Add coconut and coriander seeds and cook, stirring, until coconut is lightly golden, 2–3 minutes. Let cool slightly, then transfer to a spice grinder and grind to a fine powder.
4. In a large frying pan, heat oil and butter over high heat. Add cinnamon and cloves and cook, stirring, until fragrant, about 30 seconds. Add cooked lamb mixture and coconut mixture and cook, stirring and tossing, until mixture is lightly golden, 2–3 minutes. Remove from heat and toss in cilantro.
5. Taste and adjust seasoning with salt if necessary. Transfer to a serving dish, sprinkle with garam masala and serve immediately.

Serves 4–6 with rice and 1 or more accompaniments
Serves 6–8 with rice, 1 or more accompaniments, 1 vegetarian main dish, and 1 chicken or seafood main dish

Fish in mustard oil with five spices
Maachher jhole

1¹/₂ lb (750 g) white fish fillets
such as snapper or cod, cut into
1-inch (2.5-cm) pieces
1 teaspoon ground turmeric
¹/₄ cup (2 fl oz/60 ml) mustard oil
1 teaspoon Panch Phoron (page 31)
1 dried red chili
2 Indian bay leaves
¹/₄ teaspoon powdered asafetida
1¹/₂ teaspoons cumin seeds,
ground in spice grinder
1¹/₂ teaspoons chili powder
¹/₂ lb (250 g) medium potatoes,
cut into 1-inch (2.5-cm) pieces
¹/₂ lb (250 g) zucchini (courgettes),
cut into 1-inch (2.5-cm) pieces
1 cup (8 fl oz/250 ml) water
1 teaspoon sugar
1 teaspoon salt

Steamed Basmati Rice (page 141) or
Coconut Rice (page 85) for serving
Chickpea Chutney (page 112), Fava
Beans in Tamarind Sauce (page 113),
Mango Pickle, Andhra Pradesh Style
(page 112) and/or Home-Style Okra
Pickle (page 113) for serving

The best way to describe this dish is Bengali soul food. It is a dinnertime staple in every Bengali household.

1. In a bowl, combine fish and turmeric and toss well to combine. Set aside.
2. In a large frying pan, heat oil over high heat. When it starts to smoke, reduce heat to medium–high. Working in batches, add fish and cook, turning once, until golden, 3–4 minutes. Remove fish from pan and set aside.
3. Add panch phoron to pan over medium heat and cook, stirring, until it starts to caramelize. Add dried chili, bay leaves, asafetida, cumin, chili powder, potatoes and zucchini and cook, stirring, for 2–3 minutes. Add water and bring to a simmer. Reduce heat to low, cover and cook until potatoes and zucchini are tender, 10–15 minutes.
4. Stir in sugar and salt and return fish to pan. Cook, stirring, until fish is heated through, 2–3 minutes. Transfer to a serving dish and serve hot.

Serves 4–6 with rice and 1 or more accompaniments
Serves 6–8 with rice, 1 or more accompaniments, 1 vegetarian main dish, and 1 chicken or lamb main dish

Fish in mustard oil with five spices (front), mango pickle, Andhra Pradesh style (back left), home-style okra pickle (back right)

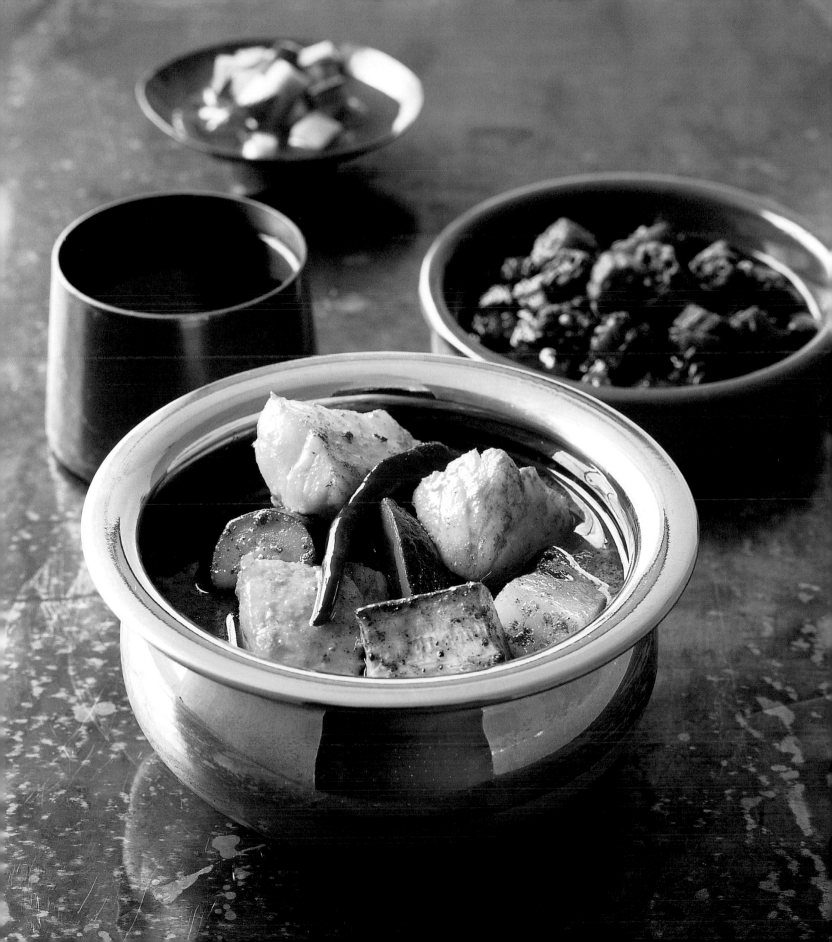

Shrimp with spinach
Thotikura petakaya

1/2 cup (4 fl oz/125 ml) vegetable oil
1/2 teaspoon black or brown mustard seeds
1 yellow (brown) onion, minced
1 teaspoon grated fresh ginger
1 teaspoon minced garlic
1 teaspoon salt
1/4 teaspoon ground turmeric
2 lb (1 kg) medium shrimp (prawns), peeled and deveined
1 lb (500 g) spinach, stems removed and chopped
4 fresh mild long green chilies, slit lengthwise

Steamed Basmati Rice (page 141) or Coconut Rice (page 85) for serving
Chickpea Chutney (page 112), Fava Beans in Tamarind Sauce (page 113), Mango Pickle, Andhra Pradesh Style (page 112) and/or Home-Style Okra Pickle (page 113) for serving

Here is my adaptation of a traditional East Indian dish that typically combines shrimp and amaranth greens.

1. In a large frying pan, heat oil over medium heat. Add mustard seeds and cook, stirring, until they pop, 2–3 minutes. Stir in onion, ginger, garlic, salt and turmeric and cook over low heat, stirring often, until onion is softened, 10–15 minutes.
2. Raise heat to high and add shrimp and spinach. Cook, stirring and tossing, until shrimp are just cooked and spinach is wilted, 3–4 minutes. Toss in chilies.
3. Taste and adjust seasoning with salt if necessary. Transfer to a serving dish and serve hot.

Serves 4–6 with rice and 1 or more accompaniments
Serves 6–8 with rice, 1 or more accompaniments, 1 vegetarian main dish, and 1 chicken or lamb main dish

Fried fish with tomatoes
Yara chapa

1 teaspoon coriander seeds
1 teaspoon cumin seeds
4 large, ripe tomatoes, roughly
chopped
4 yellow (brown) onions, halved and
thinly sliced
2 teaspoons minced garlic
1 teaspoon grated fresh ginger
1/2 teaspoon ground turmeric
2 teaspoons salt
1 1/2 lb (750 g) white fish fillets such as
snapper or cod, cut into
2-inch (5-cm) pieces
1 cup (8 fl oz/250 ml) vegetable oil
1 1/2 cups (12 fl oz/375 ml) water
1 teaspoon chili powder
3 potatoes, about 6 oz (180 g) each,
peeled and cut lengthwise into slices
1/4 inch (6 mm) thick

Steamed Basmati Rice (page 141) or
Coconut Rice (page 85) for serving
Chickpea Chutney (page 112), Fava
Beans in Tamarind Sauce (page 113),
Mango Pickle, Andhra Pradesh Style
(page 112) and/or Home-Style Okra
Pickle (page 113) for serving

Here is a modestly sophisticated version of home-style fried fish.

1. In a spice grinder, combine coriander and cumin seeds and grind to a fine powder. Transfer ground spices to a food processor. Add tomatoes, onions, garlic and ginger and process until well combined. Set aside.
2. In a bowl, combine turmeric and 1 teaspoon salt. Add fish and toss to coat fish evenly. Set aside for 5 minutes.
3. In a large frying pan, heat oil over medium–high heat. When hot, working in batches, add fish and cook, turning once, until golden brown, 2–3 minutes. Using a slotted spoon, transfer to paper towels to drain.
4. Drain off half of oil from pan. Heat remaining oil over medium heat. Carefully stir in tomato mixture, water and chili powder and bring to a simmer. Add potatoes and simmer, uncovered, until potatoes are just tender, 10–15 minutes.
5. Return fish to pan and cook until heated through, 2–3 minutes. Stir in remaining 1 teaspoon salt.
6. Transfer to a serving dish and serve hot.

Serves 4–6 with rice and 1 or more accompaniments
Serves 6–8 with rice, 1 or more accompaniments, 1 vegetarian main dish, and 1 chicken or lamb main dish

Andhra-style cucumber dal
Dosakai pappu

2 cups (14 oz/440 g) split yellow lentils
7¹/₂ cups (60 fl oz/1.8 L) water
1 tablespoon vegetable oil
¹/₂ teaspoon black or brown mustard seeds
¹/₂ teaspoon split white lentils (optional)
1 dried red chili, broken into small pieces
1 tablespoon chili powder
¹/₂ teaspoon ground turmeric
¹/₄ teaspoon powdered asafetida
1 small English (hothouse) or Lebanese cucumber, peeled and cut into small pieces
1 tablespoon tamarind concentrate
1 teaspoon salt
chili powder for serving (optional)
pappadams for serving (optional)

Steamed Basmati Rice (page 141) or Coconut Rice (page 85) for serving
Chickpea Chutney (page 112), Fava Beans in Tamarind Sauce (page 113), Mango Pickle, Andhra Pradesh Style (page 112) and/or Home-Style Okra Pickle (page 113) for serving

1. Rinse split yellow lentils. In a saucepan, combine lentils and 7 cups (56 fl oz/1.75 L) water, cover and bring to a boil over medium–high heat. Reduce heat to medium–low, uncover and simmer, stirring often, until lentils break down and mixture is like a thick mash, about 50 minutes. Set aside.
2. In a large frying pan, heat oil over medium heat. Add mustard seeds and cook, stirring, until they pop, 2–3 minutes. Stir in split white lentils if using and dried chili and cook, stirring, for 1 minute. Add chili powder, turmeric and asafetida and cook, stirring, for 1 minute. Stir in cucumber, tamarind and remaining ¹/₂ cup (4 fl oz/125 ml) water, reduce heat to low and simmer until cucumber is tender, 2–3 minutes.
3. Stir cooked lentils and salt into pan. Taste and adjust seasoning with salt if necessary. Stir over medium heat until warmed through. Transfer to a serving dish, sprinkle with extra chili powder if desired, and serve hot, with pappadams, if desired.

Serves 4–6 (vegetarian menu) with rice, 1 or more accompaniments, and 1 vegetarian main dish
Serves 4–6 (meat menu) with rice, 1 or more accompaniments, and 1 chicken, lamb or seafood main dish
Serves 6–8 (vegetarian menu) with rice, 1 or more accompaniments, and 2 other vegetarian main dishes
Serves 6–8 (meat menu) with rice, 1 or more accompaniments, 1 vegetarian main dish, and 1 chicken, lamb or seafood main dish

Andhra-style cucumber dal served with pappadams, home-style okra pickle and chickpea chutney

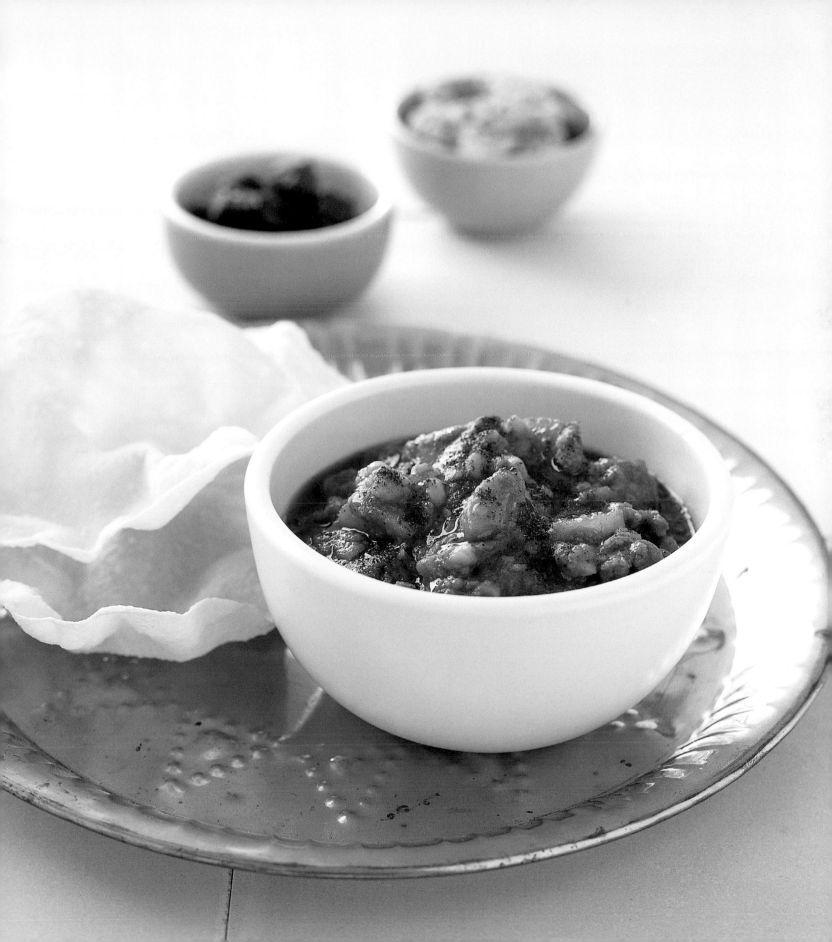

Mixed-vegetable stew
Mukkala pulusu

1 large or 2 medium orange-fleshed sweet potatoes (kumara), 10 oz (300 g), peeled and cut into 1-inch (2.5-cm) pieces
²/₃ -lb (300-g) piece pumpkin, seeds removed, peeled, and cut into 1-inch (2.5-cm) pieces
2 tablespoons vegetable oil
5 oz (150 g) okra, trimmed
1 cup (8 fl oz/250 ml) hot water
1 tablespoon tamarind concentrate
2 teaspoons chili powder
¹/₄ teaspoon ground turmeric
10 fresh curry leaves
1 teaspoon salt
1 tablespoon grated jaggery or dark brown sugar
8 oz (250 g) zucchini (courgettes) or eggplant (aubergine), cut into 1-inch (2.5-cm) pieces
¹/₂ teaspoon black or brown mustard seeds
¹/₂ teaspoon cumin seeds
¹/₄ teaspoon powdered asafetida

Steamed Basmati Rice (page 141) or Coconut Rice (page 85) for serving
Chickpea Chutney (page 112), Fava Beans in Tamarind Sauce (page 113), Mango Pickle, Andhra Pradesh Style (page 112) and/or Home-Style Okra Pickle (page 113) for serving

1. Bring a saucepan filled with salted water to a boil, add sweet potatoes and pumpkin and cook until tender, about 10 minutes. Drain.
2. Meanwhile, in a frying pan, heat 1 tablespoon oil over high heat. Add okra and cook, stirring often, until golden brown, 3–4 minutes. Transfer to a plate and set aside.
3. In a saucepan, stir together hot water and tamarind until well combined. Add cooked sweet potato and pumpkin, chili powder, turmeric, curry leaves, salt and jaggery or brown sugar. Bring to a simmer over medium heat and cook, uncovered, until vegetables break down and mixture is quite thick, 15–20 minutes. Add zucchini or eggplant for last 10 minutes of cooking.
4. Add okra to pan and simmer until heated through, 2–3 minutes.
5. In a small frying pan, heat remaining 1 tablespoon oil over medium heat. Add mustard seeds, cumin seeds and asafetida and cook, stirring, until seeds start to pop, 2–3 minutes. Pour over top of vegetables and serve immediately.

Serves 4–6 (vegetarian menu) with rice, 1 or more accompaniments, and Andhra-style Cucumber Dal (page 106)
Serves 4–6 (meat menu) with rice, 1 or more accompaniments, and 1 chicken, lamb or seafood main dish
Serves 6–8 (vegetarian menu) with rice, 1 or more accompaniments, Andhra-style Cucumber Dal (page 106), and 1 other vegetarian main dish
Serves 6–8 (meat menu) with rice, 1 or more accompaniments, 1 vegetarian main dish, and 1 chicken, lamb or seafood main dish

Mixed vegetables, Bengali style
Suktoni or sukto

1 teaspoon black or brown
mustard seeds
¹/₂ teaspoon caraway seeds
2 tablespoons mustard oil
2 Indian bay leaves
1¹/₂ tablespoons Panch Phoron
(page 31)
2 teaspoons grated fresh ginger
8 oz (250 g) potatoes, cut into
¹/₄-inch (6-mm) pieces
8 oz (250 g) orange-fleshed sweet
potatoes (kumara), peeled and
cut into ¹/₄-inch (6-mm) pieces
4 oz (125 g) daikon, cut into ¹/₄-inch
(6-mm pieces)
2 small green bananas, 4 oz (125 g)
total weight, peeled and cut into
¹/₄-inch (6-mm) pieces
5 oz (150 g) young, tender fava
(broad) beans, cut into ¹/₄-inch
(6-mm) pieces
1 small eggplant (aubergine),
5 oz (150 g), cut into ¹/₄ -inch
(6-mm) pieces
2 cups (16 fl oz/500 ml) water
1 teaspoon salt

Steamed Basmati Rice (page 141) or
Coconut Rice (page 85) for serving
Chickpea Chutney (page 112), Fava
Beans in Tamarind Sauce (page 113),
Mango Pickle, Andhra Pradesh Style
(page 112) and/or Home-Style Okra
Pickle (page 113) for serving

1. In a spice grinder, combine mustard seeds and caraway seeds and grind to a fine powder. Set aside.
2. In a saucepan, heat oil over medium–high heat. When it starts to smoke, reduce heat to medium. Add bay leaves and panch phoron and cook, stirring, until fragrant, 1–2 minutes. Stir in ground mustard and caraway seeds and cook, stirring, until fragrant, about 2 minutes.
3. Add ginger, potatoes, sweet potato, daikon, bananas, fava beans and eggplant to pan. Stir in water and salt and bring to a boil over medium–high heat. Reduce heat to medium, cover and simmer for 10 minutes. Uncover and continue to simmer until vegetables are tender, about 10 minutes longer.
4. Taste and adjust seasoning with salt if necessary. Transfer to a serving dish and serve hot.

Serves 4–6 (vegetarian menu) with rice, 1 or more accompaniments, and Andhra-Style Cucumber Dal (page 106)
Serves 4–6 (meat menu) with rice, 1 or more accompaniments, and 1 chicken, lamb or seafood main dish
Serves 6–8 (vegetarian menu) with rice, 1 or more accompaniments, Andhra-Style Cucumber Dal (page 106), and 1 other vegetarian main dish
Serves 6–8 (meat menu) with rice, 1 or more accompaniments, 1 vegetarian main dish, and 1 chicken, lamb or seafood main dish

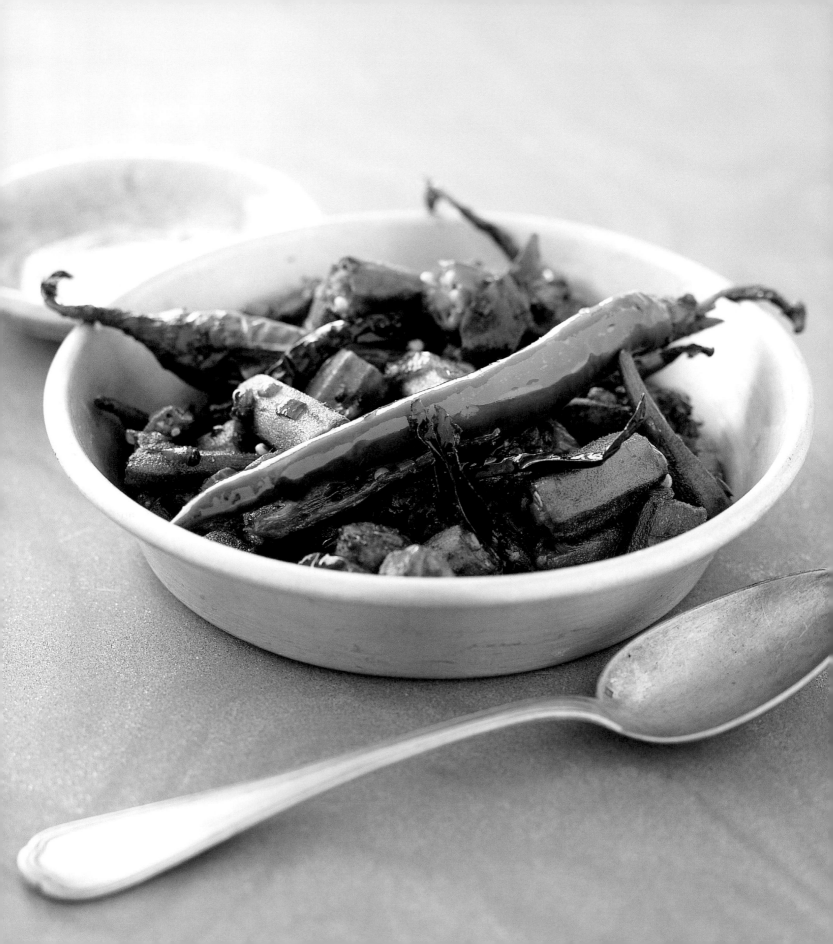

Spicy fried okra
Bendekai kura

1/3 cup (3 fl oz/90 ml) vegetable oil
4 dried red chilies
1 teaspoon black or brown mustard seeds
30 fresh curry leaves
1 lb (500 g) okra, cut into 1-inch (2.5-cm) pieces
2 yellow (brown) onions, finely chopped
3 fresh mild long green chilies, slit lengthwise
1 teaspoon salt
1 teaspoon grated jaggery or dark brown sugar
1 1/2 teaspoons coriander seeds, ground in spice grinder
1 1/2 teaspoons cumin seeds, ground in spice grinder
1 1/2 teaspoons tamarind concentrate
1/4 cup (2 fl oz/60 ml) water

Steamed Basmati Rice (page 141) or Coconut Rice (page 85) for serving
Chickpea Chutney (page 112), Fava Beans in Tamarind Sauce (page 113), Mango Pickle, Andhra Pradesh Style (page 112) for serving

1. In a large frying pan, heat oil over medium heat. Add dried chilies, mustard seeds and curry leaves and cook, stirring, until curry leaves are crisp, 3–4 minutes.
2. Add okra, onions, fresh chilies and salt to pan and cook over medium heat, stirring often, until lightly golden, 4–5 minutes.
3. Add jaggery or brown sugar, coriander and cumin to pan and cook, stirring, for 2 minutes. Stir in tamarind and water, reduce heat to low and cook, uncovered, until okra is very tender, 10–15 minutes.
4. Taste and adjust seasoning with salt if necessary. Transfer to a serving dish and serve hot.

Serves 4–6 (vegetarian menu) with rice, 1 or more accompaniments, and Andhra-style Cucumber Dal (page 106)
Serves 4–6 (meat menu) with rice, 1 or more accompaniments and 1 chicken, lamb or seafood main dish
Serves 6–8 (vegetarian menu) with rice, 1 or more accompaniments, Andhra-style Cucumber Dal (page 106), and 1 other vegetarian main dish
Serves 6–8 (meat menu) with rice, 1 or more accompaniments, 1 vegetarian main dish, and 1 chicken, lamb or seafood main dish

Accompaniments

Chickpea chutney
Pacchi senaga pappu pacchad

1/2 cup (3 1/2 oz/100 g) roasted split chickpeas
2 fresh mild long green chilies, slit lengthwise
1/2 teaspoon tamarind concentrate
3/4 cup plus 1 tablespoon (6 1/2 fl oz/200 ml) coconut cream
1 teaspoon salt

For Tempering
1 tablespoon vegetable oil
1/2 teaspoon black or brown mustard seeds
1/2 teaspoon cumin seeds
10 fresh curry leaves

An excellent accompaniment to any meal.

1. In a food processor, combine roasted split chickpeas, chilies, tamarind and coconut cream and process until smooth. Stir in salt and transfer to a serving bowl.
2. To make tempering: In a frying pan, heat oil over medium heat. Add mustard seeds and cumin and cook, stirring, until seeds start to pop, 2–3 minutes. Remove pan from heat and toss in curry leaves.
3. Pour tempering over lentil mixture. Serve warm or at room temperature. Store leftover chutney in an airtight container in refrigerator for up to 1 week.

Makes about 1 1/4 cups

Mango pickle, Andhra Pradesh style
Avakkai

1-1 1/4 cups (8–10 fl oz/250–300 ml) vegetable oil
1 clove garlic, crushed
1 tablespoon mustard powder
1-1 1/2 tablespoons chili powder
1/2 teaspoon ground turmeric
3/4 teaspoon salt
1 lb (500 g) green mangoes, unpeeled, pitted and finely chopped

An excellent accompaniment to any meal.

1. In a frying pan, heat oil over medium heat. Add garlic, mustard powder, chili powder, turmeric and salt. Cook, stirring, until fragrant, 1–2 minutes. Set aside to cool. Stir in mangoes.
2. Transfer mango mixture to a jar with a tight-fitting lid. Make sure mango mixture is completely covered with oil (if not, pour over a little extra oil). Set aside in a cool, dry place until mango pieces soften, 1–2 weeks, stirring everyday.
3. Once opened, refrigerate for up to 3–4 months. Use a clean spoon each time you remove pickle to prevent mold from forming.

Makes about 3 cups

Fava beans in tamarind sauce
Chikkudakai koora

10 oz (300 g) young, tender fava (broad) beans, cut into 1-inch (2.5-cm) pieces
1 tablespoon chickpea flour
1 teaspoon tamarind concentrate
1 teaspoon sugar
1 teaspoon chili powder
About 1 tablespoon cold water
1 tablespoon vegetable oil
1/2 teaspoon black or brown mustard seeds
1/2 teaspoon split white lentils (optional)
1 teaspoon salt

An excellent accompaniment to any meal.

1. Bring a saucepan filled with water to a boil. Add fava beans and boil until bright green, 2–3 minutes. Drain and let cool to room temperature.
2. In a small bowl, stir together chickpea flour, tamarind, sugar and chili powder until well combined. Add enough water to make a smooth paste. Set aside.
3. In a frying pan, heat oil over medium heat. Add mustard seeds and cook, stirring, until they start to pop, 2–3 minutes. Stir in lentils if using and fry until golden brown, 3–4 minutes.
4. Add cooled beans and salt to pan and cook, stirring and tossing, for 2 minutes. Add chickpea paste and cook, stirring, until well combined. Cook over medium heat, stirring, until chickpea flour is cooked and golden brown, 2–3 minutes.
5. Transfer to a serving dish and serve hot.

Serves 6–8

Variation: You can replace the fava beans with Italian flat beans.

Home-style okra pickle
Bendakai gutthi koora

3/4 cup (6 fl oz/180 ml) vegetable oil
1/3 cup (1 oz/30 g) cumin seeds
3 tablespoons chili powder
1 teaspoon salt
10 oz (300 g) okra, cut into 1/4-inch (6-mm) pieces

An excellent accompaniment to any meal.

1. In a frying pan, heat oil over medium heat. Add cumin seeds and cook, stirring, until they start to pop, 2–3 minutes.
2. Remove pan from heat and stir in chili powder and salt. Stir in okra and return pan to medium heat. Cook until okra is slightly crisp, 3–4 minutes. Remove from heat and set aside to cool.
3. Transfer okra mixture to a jar with a tight-fitting lid. Make sure okra mixture is completely covered (if not, pour over a little extra oil). Set aside in a cool, dry place for 3 days before serving.
4. Once opened, refrigerate for up to 1 month. Use a clean spoon each time you remove pickle to prevent mold from forming.

Makes about 2 cups

Desserts

Mango and pistachio ice cream
Mango and pistachio kulfi

2 ripe mangoes, about 1¹/₂ lb (750 g), peeled, pitted and coarsely chopped
1 tablespoon green cardamom pods
1 can (13 fl oz/400 ml) sweetened condensed milk
2¹/₃ cups (18 fl oz/600 ml) heavy (double) cream
3 tablespoons unsalted roasted pistachio nuts, finely chopped
Mango slices and chopped pistachio nuts for serving (optional)

This is another specialty from Nilgiri's Kitchen in Sydney.

1. In a food processor, process mango until smooth. Transfer to a large bowl.
2. In a spice grinder, grind cardamom pods to a fine powder. Stir into the mango puree.
3. Add condensed milk, cream and pistachio nuts to mango mixture and stir until well combined; do not beat or whisk. Pour mixture into an 8-cup (64-fl oz/2-L) airtight container. Cover and freeze until firm.
4. To serve, scoop into serving dishes. Top with mango and pistachio nuts, if desired. Serve immediately.

Serves 10

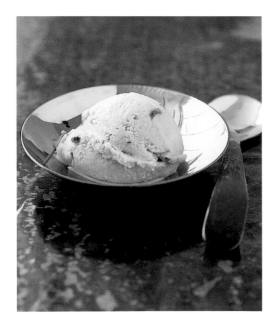

Cottage cheese dumplings in rose water and saffron syrup
Gulab jamun

For Rose Water and Saffron Syrup
4 cups (2 lb/1 kg) sugar
4 cups (32 fl oz/1 L) water
¼ teaspoon saffron threads
1 teaspoon rose water

For Dumplings
2 cups (6 oz/180 g) powdered whole milk
1 cup (5 oz/150 g) all-purpose (plain) flour
½ teaspoon ground cardamom
About 1 cup (8 fl oz/250 ml) heavy (double) cream

Vegetable oil for deep-frying

These sweet dumplings are a favorite Indian dessert. Always serve 2 or more dumplings to each diner, as it is considered rude to only offer one.

1. To make syrup: In a large saucepan, combine sugar, water, saffron and rose water. Place over low heat and stir until sugar dissolves. Keep warm over low heat.
2. To make dumplings: In a large bowl, stir together powdered milk, flour and cardamom. Add 1 cup (8 fl oz/250 ml) cream and, using your hands, gradually incorporate flour mixture into cream to form a soft dough, adding a little more cream if dough is a bit dry. Turn out dough onto a lightly floured surface and knead until mixture is very smooth and starts to become a little oily, 5–10 minutes. Shape mixture into 20 walnut-sized balls, making sure surface of each ball is very smooth.
3. Pour oil to a depth of 4 inches (10 cm) into a large, deep saucepan and heat to 350°F (180°C) on a deep-frying thermometer. Working in batches, slip dumplings into hot oil and fry, occasionally stirring gently with a large slotted spoon (do not mar surface of dumplings), until uniformly golden brown, 3–5 minutes. Using a slotted spoon, transfer to paper towels to drain for 2 minutes and then add to warm syrup. Repeat until all dumplings are fried.
4. Leave dumplings to soak in syrup for at least 30 minutes before serving.
5. Serve warm.

Serves 8

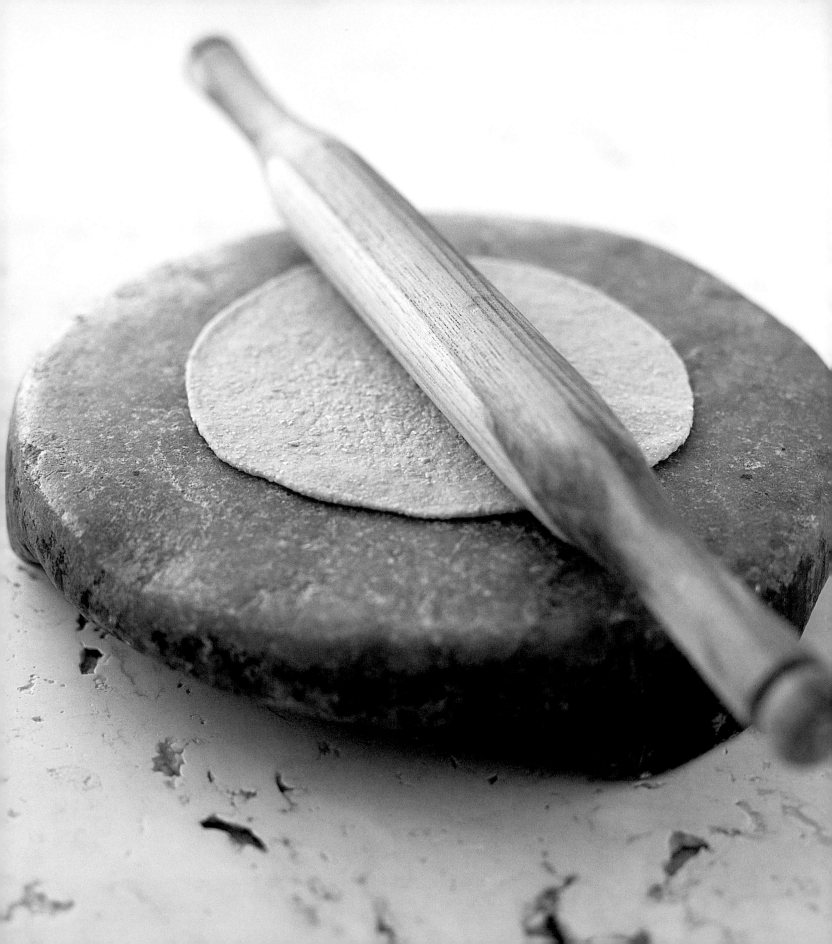

West India

Introduction

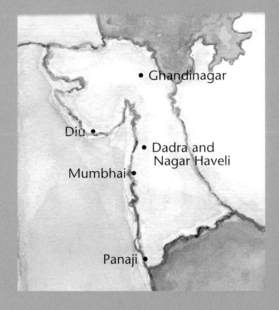

The West Region of India or Paschim Bharath is home to around 250 million Maharashtrians, Gujaratis, Parsees, Goans and some Kannadigas. The states that form the region include Gujarat, which has the longest coastline in India, Goa, Maharashtra, north Karnataka and some parts of Rajasthan.

The climate is quite dry and hot. Such states as Goa do not experience many cold days. Some parts of Maharashtra get a heavy rainfall, and its primary agricultural produce is rice. Goa, which used to be a colony of Portugal, has a strong fishing industry. The production of coconuts and coconut oil is also strong in this area. Other produce of the region includes peanuts, sugarcane and dates.

The state of Gujarat has a very high standard of living. Thriving businesses include the petrochemical and textile industries. Wildlife includes the large Asiatic lion, wild asses, flamingos, sloth bears, snakes (particularly in Goa) and foxes.

This region is also the home of some of the hottest and best-known spices, which are liberally used in the dishes of the region. Food from this region reflects the history, beliefs and lifestyle of the people. The Hindus of Goa use "kokum" as a souring agent and the Muslims use tamarind, while the Christians use vinegar, which some believe was introduced to West India by the Portuguese. Maharashtrian food, on the other hand, is rich and reflects the wealth of the Patil community, who are the landlords of this region.

There is an abundance of coconut and seafood, both of which are used widely in this region, along with some common spices, such as cassia, clove, cardamom and bay leaf (tez pat).

A distinctive flavor from this region is the Balchao Masala, which is a simple spice mixture featuring two types of chilies, vinegars, black peppercorns, coriander seeds, turmeric, garlic and ginger. An array of dishes can be made using this mixture – a golden opportunity to let your imagination run wild!

This region is also the home of the famous Kutchi Biriyani (a type of Muslim Biryani).

Enjoy the flexibility and delightful richness of West Indian cooking!

Starters

Onion pakoras
Kanda vada

2 bunches scallions (shallots/spring onions), thinly sliced
2 fresh mild long green chilies, thinly sliced
1/4 cup (1/3 oz/10 g) chopped fresh cilantro (fresh coriander)
1 teaspoon minced garlic
1 teaspoon grated fresh ginger
1 teaspoon salt
1/2 teaspoon chili powder
1/2 teaspoon ground turmeric
1/2 cup (21/2 oz/75 g) chickpea flour, or as needed
Vegetable oil for deep-frying
Mango Chutney (page 140) for serving

Also known as onion bajji, the popularity of this starter extends beyond India's western region.

1. In a bowl, stir together scallions, chilies, cilantro, garlic, ginger, salt, chili powder and turmeric. Add 1/2 cup (21/2 oz/75 g) flour and mix until well combined. Mixture should bind together; if it doesn't, add a little more flour. Do not add water.
2. Pour oil to a depth of 2 inches (5 cm) into a large, deep frying pan and heat to 350°F (180°C) on a deep-frying thermometer. While oil is heating, shape tablespoonfuls of scallion mixture into thin, flat rounds. You should have 16 rounds.
3. When oil is ready, slip 4 or 5 rounds into hot oil and cook, turning occasionally, until golden brown and crispy, 2–3 minutes. Using a slotted spoon, transfer rounds to paper towels to drain. Repeat with remaining rounds.
4. Serve hot with chutney.

Serves 4 as a starter
Serves 6–8 as a starter with 1 other starter
Serves 8–10 as a starter with all 3 starters

Onion pakoras (center), mango chutney (front right), spiced fish (back right)

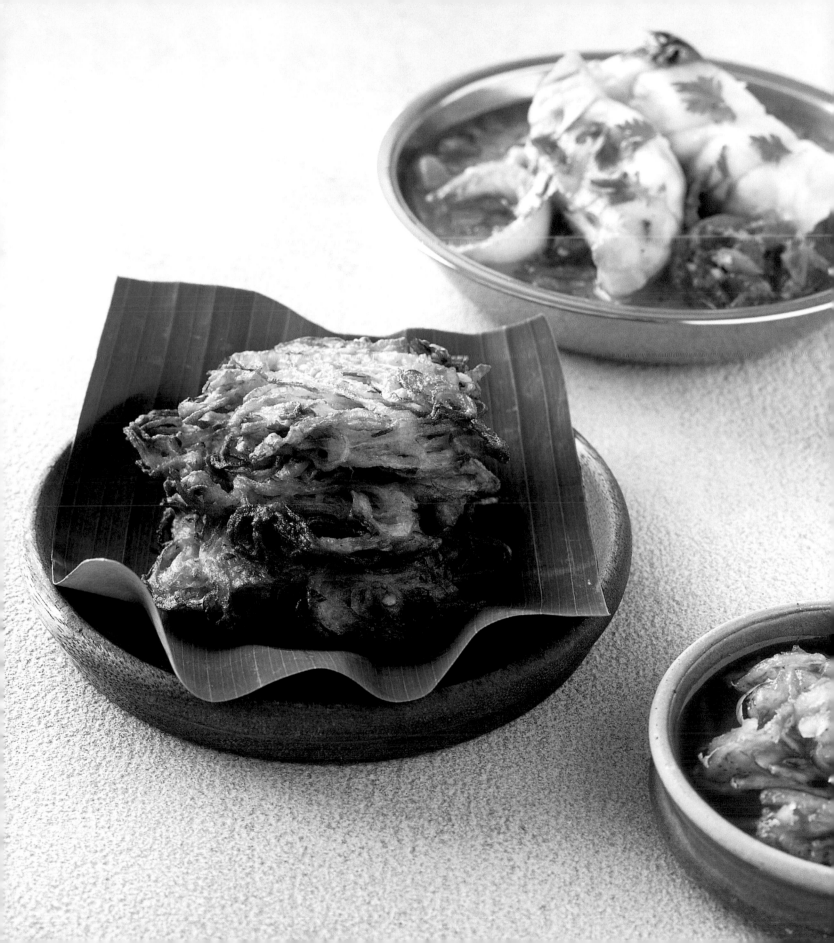

Spiced fish
Masalechi masoli

1 tablespoon minced garlic
1 tablespoon grated fresh ginger
1 fresh mild long green chili,
finely chopped
1 teaspoon salt
2 tablespoons desiccated coconut
1/4 cup (2 fl oz/60 ml) vegetable oil
2 yellow (brown) onions, sliced into
thick rings
2 ripe tomatoes, chopped
1 teaspoon Nilgiri's Garam Masala
(page 28)
1 teaspoon coriander seeds, ground in
spice grinder
1/2 teaspoon ground turmeric
1 lb (500 g) white fish fillets such
as snapper or cod, cut into
1-inch (2.5-cm) thick slices
1/4 cup (1/3 oz/10 g) chopped fresh
cilantro (fresh coriander)

The fishermen's community of the west coast makes this simple, tasty dish.

1. In a bowl, stir together garlic, ginger, chili, salt and coconut.
2. In a heavy-bottomed frying pan, heat oil over medium heat. Add onions, tomatoes, garam masala, coriander, turmeric and coconut mixture and cook uncovered, stirring often, until onions start to soften, 7–8 minutes.
3. Place fish on top of cooked onion mixture, reduce heat to low, cover and cook until fish is just cooked and flakes when tested with a fork, 8–10 minutes.
4. Transfer to a serving dish and sprinkle with cilantro. Serve hot.

Serves 4 as a starter
Serves 6–8 as a starter with 1 other starter
Serves 8–10 as a starter with all 3 starters

Spiced lamb chops
Lamb chaps masaledar

3 tablespoons vegetable oil
1 yellow (brown) onion, halved and thinly sliced
1 teaspoon salt
1 tablespoon minced garlic
2 teaspoons grated fresh ginger
3 fresh mild long green chilies, finely chopped
$1/2$ teaspoon ground turmeric
$1/2$ teaspoon chili powder
8 lamb rib chops (cutlets), about 1 lb (500 g) total weight
$1/2$ cup (4 oz/125 g) plain whole-milk yogurt
$1/2$ cup (4 fl oz/125 ml) water
2 tablespoons desiccated coconut
1 teaspoon Nilgiri's Garam Masala (page 28)

From the heartland of Maharashtra, this dish is popular with the farming community.

1. In a large frying pan, heat oil over medium–low heat. Add onion and salt and cook uncovered, stirring occasionally, until onion is dark golden brown, 20–25 minutes. Raise heat to high, stir in garlic, ginger and chilies and cook, stirring, for 2 minutes.
2. Stir in turmeric and chili powder, add lamb chops and cook, turning once, until browned, 1–2 minutes. Meanwhile, in a bowl, whisk together yogurt, water and coconut. When chops are ready, add yogurt mixture to pan and cook, uncovered, until lamb is cooked, about 5 minutes.
3. Transfer to a serving plate and sprinkle with garam masala. Serve hot.

Serves 4 as a starter
Serves 6–8 as a starter with 1 other starter
Serves 8–10 as a starter with all 3 starters

Main Dishes

Chicken with cinnamon and coconut
Chicken shakuti

For Shakuti Masala
8 dried Kashmiri red chilies, broken into small pieces
2-inch (5-cm) piece cinnamon stick, broken into small pieces
1 tablespoon coriander seeds
1 teaspoon fenugreek seeds
6 whole cloves
5 black peppercorns
4 green cardamom pods
1/2 teaspoon cumin seeds
2 teaspoons unsalted roasted peanuts, roughly chopped
1 teaspoon ground turmeric
1 can (13 fl oz/400 ml) coconut cream

2 tablespoons vegetable oil
4 yellow (brown) onions, halved and thinly sliced
2 teaspoons salt
1/4 cup (2 fl oz/60 ml) water
1 whole chicken, 3 lb (1.5 kg), cut into 10 pieces, or 2 lb (1 kg) chicken pieces
Juice of 1 lime
Lime wedges for serving (optional)

Steamed Basmati Rice (page 141) and/or Home-style Bread (page 141) for serving
Mango Chutney (page 140) and/or Carrot and Roast Peanut Relish (page 140) for serving

Chicken with cinnamon and coconut (front),
Carrot and roast peanut relish (back left),
steamed basmati rice (back center)

This is a specialty of cooks in Goa.

1. To make masala: In a spice grinder, combine chilies, cinnamon, coriander, fenugreek, cloves, peppercorns, cardamom and cumin and grind to a fine powder. Transfer to a small food processor, add peanuts and turmeric and process to combine. Add coconut cream and process until well combined.
2. In a large, heavy-bottomed saucepan, heat oil over medium–low heat. Add onions and salt and cook uncovered, stirring occasionally, until onions are softened, 10–15 minutes. Raise heat to medium, add masala and water and cook, stirring, until sauce comes to a simmer.
3. Add chicken pieces to pan and simmer, uncovered, until chicken is cooked through and tender, about 20 minutes.
4. Remove pan from heat and stir in lime juice. Transfer to serving dish and serve hot.

Serves 4–6 with rice and/or bread, and 1 or 2 accompaniments
Serves 6–8 with rice and/or bread, 1 or 2 accompaniments, 1 vegetarian main dish, and 1 lamb or seafood main dish

Note: Use regular dried red chilies if Kashmiri chilies are unavailable. Reduce the number to 4 dried red chilies, as Kashmiri chilies are milder.

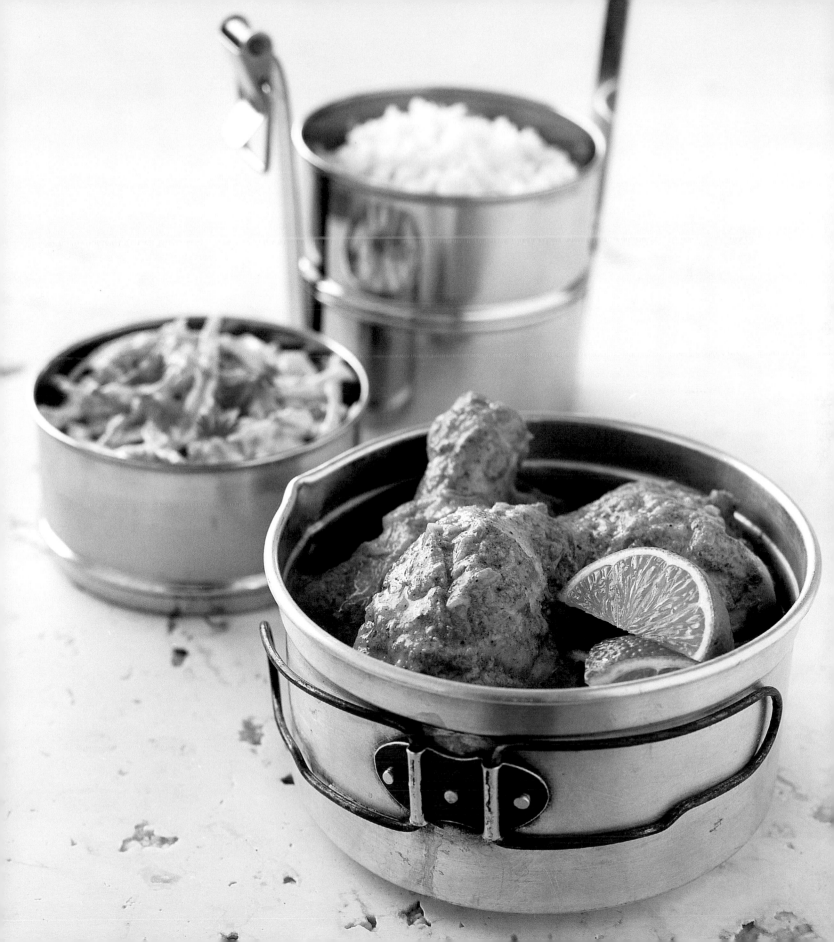

Chicken with cauliflower

Kheema aur phool-gobi

2 yellow (brown) onions, roughly chopped
2 tablespoons minced garlic
1 teaspoon grated fresh ginger
4 tablespoons vegetable oil
1 teaspoon Nilgiri's Garam Masala (page 28)
1 teaspoon ground turmeric
8 oz (250 g) ground (minced) chicken
2 tablespoons unsalted roasted cashew nuts
2 tablespoons unsalted roasted peanuts
2–3 tablespoons hot water
1 cauliflower, about 1³/4 lb (875 g)
4 ripe tomatoes, chopped
1 teaspoon salt
1 teaspoon chili powder
1 can (13 fl oz/400 ml) coconut milk
1 tablespoon slivered blanched almonds, toasted
Chopped fresh cilantro (fresh coriander) for garnish

Steamed Basmati Rice (page 141) and/or Home-style Bread (page 141) for serving
Mango Chutney (page 140) and/or Carrot and Roast Peanut Relish (page 140) for serving

This recipe, from Nilgiri's restaurant, is a specialty of the Marathas.

1. In a small food processor, combine onions, garlic and ginger and process until finely chopped. In a heavy-bottomed saucepan, heat 2 tablespoons oil over medium heat. Add half of onion mixture and cook, stirring often, until golden brown, 3–4 minutes. Add garam masala and 1/2 teaspoon turmeric and cook, stirring, until fragrant, 1–2 minutes.
2. Raise heat to high, add chicken and cook until chicken changes color, 2–3 minutes. Remove pan from heat and set aside to cool slightly.
3. Transfer chicken mixture to food processor, add cashew nuts and peanuts and process until well combined. Add enough hot water to process to a fine paste.
4. Cut florets from cauliflower, keeping stalks short. In saucepan, heat remaining 2 tablespoons oil over medium heat. Add remaining onion mixture and cook, stirring, until golden brown, 2–3 minutes. Stir in tomatoes, salt, chili powder and remaining 1/2 teaspoon turmeric and cook until tomatoes break down, about 10 minutes.
5. Stir coconut milk and chicken mixture into pan. Place cauliflower in pan, heads down. Cover and cook over low heat, turning cauliflower florets once, until cauliflower is tender, 15–20 minutes.
6. Taste and adjust seasoning with salt if necessary. Transfer to serving dish and top with almonds and cilantro. Serve hot.

Serves 4–6 with rice and/or bread and 1 or 2 accompaniments
Serves 6–8 with rice and/or bread, 1 or 2 accompaniments, 1 vegetarian main dish, and 1 lamb or seafood main dish

Sour-hot chicken curry
Chicken amotik

4–6 dried Kashmiri chilies, broken into small pieces
$1/2$ teaspoon cumin seeds
$1/2$ teaspoon black peppercorns
1 tablespoon minced garlic
2 teaspoons grated fresh ginger
2 teaspoons tamarind concentrate
About 1 tablespoon white vinegar
2 tablespoons vegetable oil
2 yellow (brown) onions, halved and thinly sliced
1 teaspoon salt
2 lb (1 kg) skinless, boneless chicken thighs, trimmed of fat and cut into 1-inch (2.5-cm) pieces
$1/3$ cup (3 fl oz/90ml) water

Steamed Basmati Rice (page 141) or Coconut Rice (page 85) and/or Home-style Bread (page 141) for serving
Mango Chutney (page 140) and/or Carrot and Roast Peanut Relish (page 140) for serving

This is the second most popular dish at Sydney's Nilgiri's restaurant, next only to Shrimp Balchao (page 130).

1. In a spice grinder, combine chilies, cumin and peppercorns and grind to a fine powder. Transfer to a small bowl. Add garlic, ginger, tamarind and enough vinegar to form a paste.
2. In a heavy-bottomed saucepan, heat oil over medium–low heat. Add onions and salt and cook uncovered, stirring occasionally, until onions are softened, 10–15 minutes.
3. Raise heat to high and add spice mixture. Cook, stirring, until fragrant, 2–3 minutes. Add chicken and cook, turning once, until browned, 2–3 minutes. Pour water over chicken. Reduce heat to low, cover and cook until chicken is cooked through and tender, 10–15 minutes.
4. Transfer to serving dish and serve hot.

Serves 4–6 with rice and/or bread and 1 or 2 accompaniments
Serves 6–8 with rice and/or bread, 1 or 2 accompaniments, 1 vegetarian main dish, and 1 lamb or seafood main dish

Goan-style lamb
Gosht baffad

6 dried red chilies, broken into small pieces
2 teaspoons cumin seeds
2 teaspoons black peppercorns
6 whole cloves
1 cinnamon stick, 3 inches (7.5 cm) long
6 green cardamom pods
1^1/$_2$ tablespoons minced garlic
1 teaspoon grated fresh ginger
1 tablespoon ground turmeric
^{1}/$_4$ teaspoon tamarind concentrate
2 lb (1 kg) boneless lamb shoulder (blade), cut into 1-inch (2.5-cm) pieces
2 tablespoons vegetable oil

Steamed Basmati Rice (page 141) or Coconut Rice (page 85) and/or Home-style Bread (page 141) for serving
Mango Chutney (page 140) and/or Carrot and Roast Peanut Relish (page 140) for serving

Popular with both the Parsees and the Goans, this dish is also good made with lamb rib chops. You may want to try making it with goat as well.

1. In a spice grinder, combine chilies, cumin, peppercorns, cloves, cinnamon and cardamom and grind to a fine powder. Transfer spices to a small bowl. Stir in garlic, ginger, turmeric and tamarind to make a masala.
2. In a bowl, combine lamb and masala and stir to coat lamb evenly. Cover and set aside for 1 hour to marinate.
3. In a heavy-bottomed saucepan, heat oil over high heat. Add half of lamb and cook, turning as necessary, until well browned, 2–3 minutes. Remove meat from pan. Repeat with remaining lamb. Return all lamb to pan, reduce heat to low, cover and cook until lamb is tender, 45–60 minutes.
4. Transfer to a serving dish and serve hot.

Serves 4–6 with rice and/or bread and 1 or 2 accompaniments
Serves 6–8 with rice and/or bread, 1 or 2 accompaniments, 1 vegetarian main dish, and 1 chicken or seafood main dish

Variation: You can replace the lamb with beef. Use boneless beef chuck (neck) and increase cooking time to 1–1^1/$_2$ hours.

Lamb pulao
Kheema pullao

2¹/₂ cups (1 lb/500 g) basmati rice
3 tablespoons vegetable oil
3 yellow (brown) onions, halved and thinly sliced
1¹/₂ teaspoons salt or to taste
1 cinnamon stick, 3 inches (7.5 cm) long, broken into pieces
6 whole cloves
3 brown cardamom pods
3 green cardamom pods
2 bay leaves
2 tablespoons minced garlic
1¹/₂ tablespoons grated fresh ginger
1 tablespoon coriander seeds, ground in spice grinder
1¹/₂ teaspoons ground turmeric
2 fresh small red serrano or bird's eye chilies, finely chopped (optional)
¹/₄ cup (1 oz/30 g) desiccated coconut
1¹/₃ lb (650 g) ground (minced) lamb
1 cup (8 oz/250 g) plain whole-milk yogurt, whisked until smooth
3³/₄ cups (30 fl oz/900 ml) vegetable stock
3 eggs, hard-boiled, peeled and quartered
1¹/₂ teaspoons Nilgiri's Garam Masala (page 28)
Leaves from ¹/₂ bunch fresh mint, chopped
Leaves from ¹/₄ bunch fresh cilantro (fresh coriander), chopped

Home-style Bread (page 141) for serving
Mango Chutney and/or Carrot and Roast Peanut Relish (page 140) for serving

Here is a Maharashtrian version of ground lamb and rice cooked together.

1. Rinse rice under cold running water until water runs clear. Place in a bowl and cover with plenty of water. Set aside to soak for 20 minutes.
2. In a heavy-bottomed saucepan, heat oil over medium–low heat. Add onions and salt and cook uncovered, stirring occasionally, until onions are dark golden brown, 20–25 minutes.
3. Raise heat to high and add cinnamon, cloves, brown and green cardamom and bay leaves. Cook, stirring, until fragrant, 1–2 minutes. Add garlic, ginger, coriander, turmeric, chilies if using and coconut to pan and cook, stirring, for 2 minutes. Add lamb and yogurt and cook, stirring occasionally, until lamb changes color, 2–3 minutes.
4. Add stock to pan and bring to a boil. Drain rice and add to pan. Reduce heat to low, cover and cook for 10 minutes. Remove from heat and set aside, covered, for 10 minutes.
5. Toss eggs and garam masala into rice until evenly distributed. Transfer to a serving dish and sprinkle with mint and cilantro. Serve immediately.

Serves 4–6 with bread and 1 or 2 accompaniments
Serves 6–8 with bread, 1 or 2 accompaniments, 1 vegetarian main dish, and 1 chicken or seafood main dish

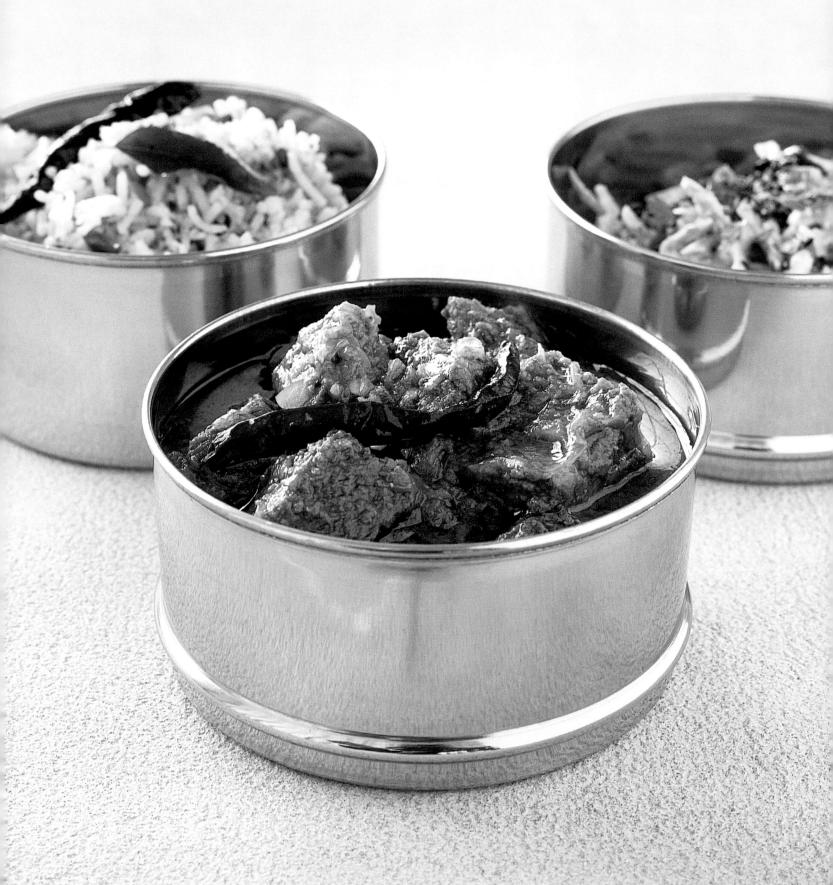

Beef assado
Bife assado

4 fresh mild long green chilies
1 tablespoon minced garlic
1 teaspoon grated fresh ginger
2 teaspoons ground turmeric
1/4 teaspoon cracked black pepper
2 teaspoons white vinegar
2 lb (1 kg) boneless stewing beef
such as chuck steak, cut into
1-inch (2.5-cm) pieces
3 tablespoons vegetable oil
3 yellow (brown) onions, halved and
thinly sliced
1 teaspoon salt
1 dried red chili

Steamed Basmati Rice (page 141) or
Coconut Rice (page 85) and/or Home-
style Bread (page 141) for serving
Mango Chutney (page 140) and/or
Carrot and Roast Peanut Relish (page
140) for serving

Gerry Mudar, a Goan chef at Nilgiri's, developed this recipe, which illustrates the Portuguese influence on Goan food by using vinegar.

1. In a small food processor, combine fresh chilies, garlic and ginger and process until chilies are finely chopped. Add turmeric, pepper and vinegar and process until a paste forms. Transfer paste to a bowl, add meat and toss well to coat meat evenly. Cover and set aside for 3 hours to marinate.
2. In a heavy-bottomed ovenproof saucepan, heat oil over medium–low heat. Add onions and salt and cook uncovered, stirring occasionally, until onions are softened, 10–15 minutes. Preheat oven to 300°F (150°C/Gas 2).
3. Raise heat to high, add half of beef and cook, stirring, until well browned, 2–3 minutes. Remove beef and onions from pan. Repeat with remaining beef. Return all beef to pan and add dried chili.
4. Cover, place in oven and cook until beef is very tender, about 1 1/2 hours.
5. Taste and adjust seasoning with salt if necessary. Transfer to a serving dish and serve hot.

Serves 4–6 with rice and/or bread and 1 or 2 accompaniments
Serves 6–8 with rice and/or bread, 1 or 2 accompaniments, 1 vegetarian main dish, and 1 chicken or seafood main dish

Variation: You can substitute lamb cut from leg for the beef.

Beef assado (front), coconut rice (back left), carrot and roast peanut relish (back right)

Shrimp balchao

1/3 cup (3 fl oz/90 ml) vegetable oil
1 yellow (brown) onion, halved and thinly sliced
1 teaspoon salt
1 recipe Balchao Masala (page 31)
2 lb (1 kg) medium shrimp (prawns), peeled and deveined
Juice of 1 lemon
Chopped fresh cilantro (fresh coriander) for serving

Steamed Basmati Rice (page 141) or Coconut Rice (page 85) and/or Home-style Bread (page 141) for serving
Mango Chutney (page 140) and/or Carrot and Roast Peanut Relish (page 140) for serving

I learned this recipe from chef AC Alex at the Taj Residency in Bangalore, and it was by far the most popular dish at the Southern Comfort restaurant, also in Bangalore.

1. In a large frying pan, heat oil over medium–low heat. Add onion and salt and cook uncovered, stirring occasionally, until onions are dark golden brown, 20–25 minutes.
2. Raise heat to medium, add balchao masala and cook, stirring, until fragrant, about 2 minutes. Raise heat to high, add shrimp and cook, stirring and tossing, until shrimp are just cooked, 3–4 minutes.
3. Remove pan from heat and stir in lemon juice. Taste and adjust seasoning with salt if necessary. Transfer to a serving dish and sprinkle with cilantro. Serve hot.

Serves 4–6 with rice and/or bread and 1 or 2 accompaniments
Serves 6–8 with rice and/or bread, 1 or 2 accompaniments, 1 vegetarian main dish, and 1 chicken or meat main dish

Shrimp balchao (front), home-style bread (back left), mango chutney (back right)

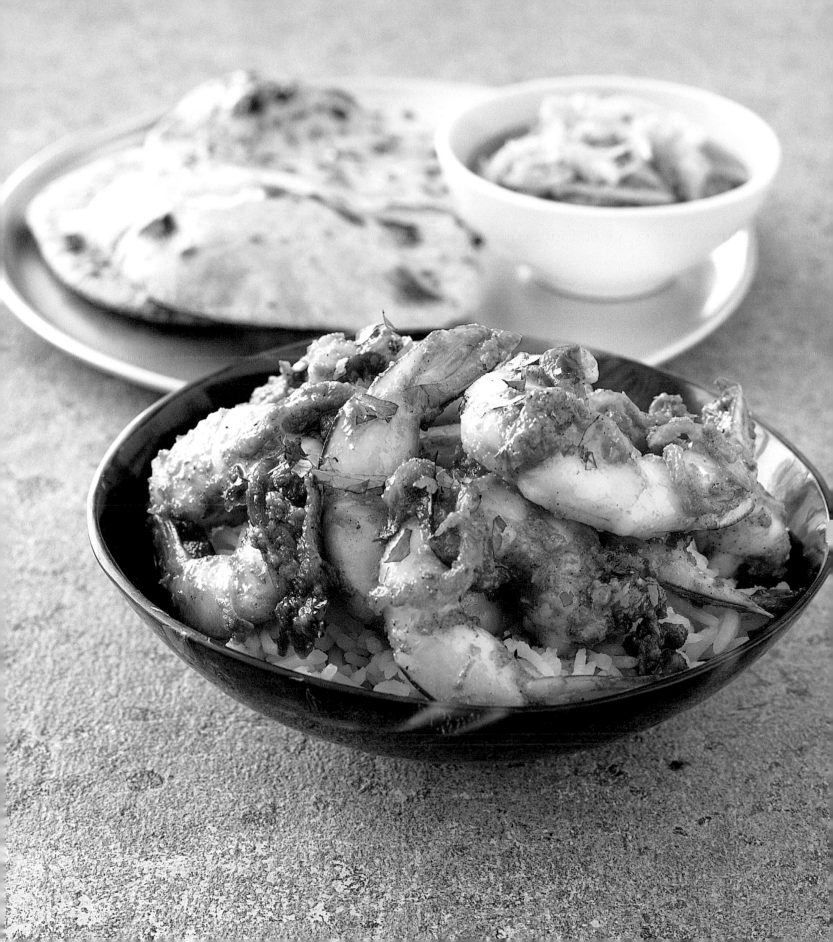

Yellow fish curry
Caldine

¹/₄ teaspoon cumin seeds
1-inch (2.5-cm) piece fresh ginger,
peeled and roughly chopped
3 cloves garlic
1 teaspoon ground turmeric
1 can (13 fl oz/400 ml) coconut cream
2 tablespoons vegetable oil
1 yellow (brown) onion, chopped
1 teaspoon salt
2 fresh mild long green chilies,
slit lengthwise
1¹/₂ lb (750 g) white fish fillets such
as snapper or cod, cut into
2-inch (5-cm) pieces
Juice of 1 lemon

Steamed Basmati Rice (page 141)
and/or Home-style Bread (page 141)
for serving
Mango Chutney (page 140) and/or
Carrot and Roast Peanut Relish
(page 140) for serving

An absolute treat to the eyes and taste buds.

1. In a spice grinder, grind cumin seeds to a fine powder. Transfer to a food processor, add ginger, garlic and turmeric and process until roughly chopped. Add a little of the coconut cream and process to form a fine paste. Add remaining coconut cream and process to combine.
2. In a large frying pan, heat oil over medium–low heat. Add onion and salt and cook uncovered, stirring occasionally, until onion is dark golden brown, 20–25 minutes.
3. Raise heat to medium, add chilies and cook, stirring, for 2 minutes. Add spice mixture and cook, stirring, until sauce comes to a simmer. Add fish and cook until fish is just cooked and flakes when tested with a fork, 8–10 minutes.
4. Remove pan from heat and stir in lemon juice. Taste and adjust seasoning with salt if necessary. Transfer to a serving dish and serve immediately.

Serves 4–6 with rice and/or bread and 1 or 2 accompaniments
Serves 6–8 with rice and/or bread, 1 or 2 accompaniments, 1 vegetarian main dish, and 1 chicken or meat main dish

Note: This recipe is best eaten the day after it is made. Reheat gently over medium–low heat.

Sweet, sour and hot crab
Denji amotik

2¹/₂ lb (1.25 kg) soft-shell or blue
swimmer crabs (about 4 crabs)
2 tablespoons vegetable oil
1 yellow (brown) onion, halved and
thinly sliced
1 teaspoon salt
1 recipe Balchao Masala (page 31)
1 cup (8 fl oz/250 ml) coconut cream
1 teaspoon tamarind concentrate
1 teaspoon sugar

Steamed Basmati Rice (page 141)
and/or Home-style Bread (page 141)
for serving
Mango Chutney (page 140) and/or
Carrot and Roast Peanut Relish
(page 140) for serving

This crab dish is one of my favorites and is extremely easy to make.

1. Remove large top shell from each crab. Remove fibrous matter from inside crab and discard. Rinse crabs well. Using a sharp knife, cut each crab into quarters. Use a meat mallet to crack shells on the legs. This will make the meat easier to get out once cooked. Set aside.
2. In a large, deep, wide frying pan, heat oil over medium–low heat. Add onion and salt and cook uncovered, stirring often, until onion is dark golden brown, 20–25 minutes.
3. Add balchao masala and cook, stirring, until fragrant, about 2 minutes. Add crabs and cook, stirring and tossing, for 2–3 minutes. Stir in coconut cream, cover and cook, turning crab pieces occasionally, until shells turn orange-red and meat is just cooked, 15–20 minutes.
4. Remove pan from heat. Using tongs, transfer crab pieces to a plate. Stir tamarind and sugar into pan sauce. Taste and adjust seasoning with salt if necessary.
5. Return crab pieces to pan and turn to coat with hot sauce. Transfer to a serving dish and serve immediately.

Serves 4–6 with rice and/or bread and 1 or 2 accompaniments
Serves 6–8 with rice and/or bread, 1 or 2 accompaniments, 1 vegetarian main dish, and 1 chicken or meat main dish

Note: The coconut cream will curdle when the pan is covered. Don't worry; the dish is still very good.

Spiced hard-boiled eggs
Masalache ande

6 large eggs, at room temperature
1/4 cup (1 oz/30 g) desiccated coconut
1 dried red chili
3 whole cloves
1/2-inch (12-mm) piece cinnamon stick
2 teaspoons minced garlic
1/2 teaspoon ground turmeric
1/3 cup (3 fl oz/90 ml) vegetable oil
1 yellow (brown) onion, halved and thinly sliced
1 teaspoon salt
2 teaspoons tamarind concentrate
1/2 cup (4 fl oz/125 ml) water
Fresh cilantro (fresh coriander) leaves for garnish

Steamed Basmati Rice (page 141) and/or Home-style Bread (page 141) for serving
Mango Chutney (page 140) and/or Carrot and Roast Peanut Relish (page 140) for serving

1. In a small saucepan, place eggs with cold water to cover. Cover, bring to a gentle simmer, uncover and simmer for 5 minutes. Drain, rinse under cold running water and peel eggs.
2. In a spice grinder, combine coconut, chili, cloves and cinnamon and grind to a fine powder. Transfer to a bowl and stir in garlic and turmeric. Make short, shallow slits over surface of eggs. Spread paste well over eggs.
3. In a frying pan, heat oil over medium–low heat. Add onion and salt and cook uncovered, stirring often, until onions are lightly golden, 10 minutes. Raise heat to medium–high and add eggs. Cook, turning often, for 5–6 minutes, until eggs are golden brown. Add remaining paste. Cook, tossing for 2 minutes.
4. In a small bowl, stir together tamarind and water and add to pan. Stir over medium heat until sauce thickens and coats eggs, 3–4 minutes.
5. Transfer to a serving dish and sprinkle with cilantro. Serve hot.

Serves 4–6 (vegetarian menu) with rice and/or bread, 1 or 2 accompaniments, and Red Lentil Dal (page 137)
Serves 4–6 (meat menu) with rice and/or bread, 1 or 2 accompaniments, and 1 chicken, meat or seafood main dish
Serves 6–8 (vegetarian menu) with rice and/or bread, 1 or 2 accompaniments, Red Lentil Dal (page 137), and 1 other vegetarian main dish
Serves 6–8 (meat menu) with rice and/or bread, 1 or 2 accompaniments, 1 other vegetarian main dish, and 1 chicken, meat or seafood main dish

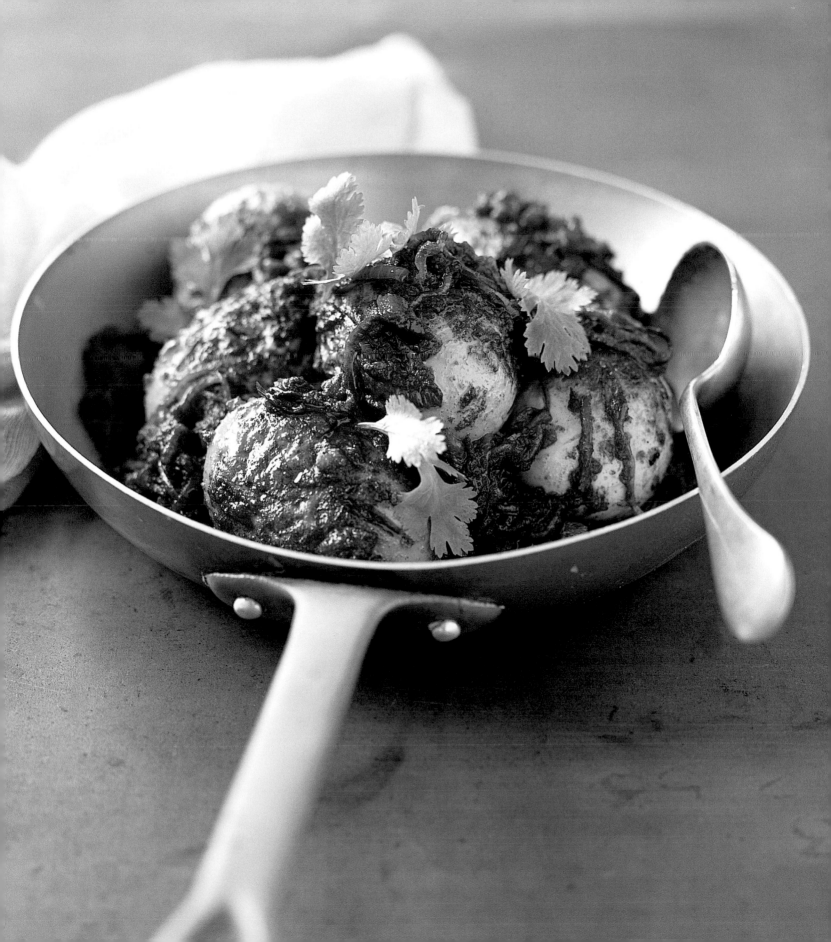

Chutney potatoes
Chatni che batate

2 lb (1 kg) red-skinned potatoes, unpeeled
1¹/₄ teaspoons cumin seeds
1 teaspoon coriander seeds
1 bunch fresh cilantro (fresh coriander), roughly chopped
4 fresh mild long green chilies, roughly chopped
1 tablespoon minced garlic
1 tablespoon grated fresh ginger
1 tablespoon desiccated coconut
1 teaspoon tamarind concentrate
¹/₂ teaspoon ground turmeric
1 teaspoon salt
1 teaspoon chili powder
3 tablespoons vegetable oil
¹/₄ teaspoon black or brown mustard seeds

Steamed Basmati Rice (page 141) and/or Home-style Bread (page 141) for serving
Mango Chutney (page 140) and/or Carrot and Roast Peanut Relish (page 140) for serving

1. In a large saucepan, combine potatoes with plenty of cold water to cover. Bring to a boil over high heat and boil, uncovered, until tender but quite firm, about 10 minutes. Drain well and set aside to cool. Cut cooled potatoes into slices 1 inch (2.5 cm) thick.
2. In a spice grinder, combine 1 teaspoon cumin seeds and coriander seeds and grind to a fine powder. Transfer to a small food processor. Add cilantro, chilies, garlic, ginger, coconut, tamarind, turmeric, salt and chili powder and process until a smooth paste forms. Transfer to a bowl, add potatoes and toss gently to coat evenly.
3. In a large frying pan, heat oil over medium heat. Add remaining ¹/₄ teaspoon cumin seeds and mustard seeds and cook, stirring, until seeds start to pop, 2–3 minutes. Add potatoes and cook, stirring occasionally, until potatoes are golden, about 10 minutes.
4. Taste and adjust seasoning with salt if necessary. Transfer to a serving dish and serve hot.

Serves 4–6 (vegetarian menu) with rice and/or bread, 1 or 2 accompaniments, and Red Lentil Dal (page 137)
Serves 4–6 (meat menu) with rice and/or bread, 1 or 2 accompaniments, and 1 chicken, meat or seafood main dish
Serves 6–8 (vegetarian menu) with rice and/or bread, 1 or 2 accompaniments, Red Lentil Dal (page 137), and 1 other vegetarian main dish
Serves 6–8 (meat menu) with rice and/or bread, 1 or 2 accompaniments, 1 other vegetarian main dish, and 1 chicken, meat or seafood main dish

Red lentil dal
Masurchi amti

1/2 cup (2 oz/60 g) desiccated coconut
1/2 cup (3 oz/90 g) unsalted roasted peanuts, finely chopped
2 cups (14 oz/440 g) red lentils
6 cups (48 fl oz/1.5 L) water
1/2 teaspoon ground turmeric
1 teaspoon tamarind concentrate
1 tablespoon finely grated jaggery
1 teaspoon salt

1 tablespoon chopped fresh cilantro (fresh coriander)

For Tempering
1 tablespoon vegetable oil
2 teaspoons Nilgiri's Garam Masala (page 28)
1 teaspoon chili powder

Steamed Basmati Rice (page 141) and/or Home-style Bread (page 141) for serving
Mango Chutney (page 140) and/or Carrot and Roast Peanut Relish (page 140) for serving

This Maharashtrian version of the Tamilian rasam also makes an excellent appetizer.

1. In a small nonstick frying pan, dry roast coconut over medium heat, stirring, until golden, 3–4 minutes. Let cool slightly, then transfer to a small food processor. Add peanuts and process to a fine paste. Set aside.
2. Rinse lentils. In a saucepan, combine lentils, water and turmeric, cover and bring to a boil over high heat. Reduce heat to medium, uncover and simmer, uncovered, until lentils break down and mixture is quite thick, 40–45 minutes.
3. Remove pan from heat and stir in coconut paste, tamarind, jaggery and salt. Taste and adjust seasoning with salt if necessary.
4. To make tempering: In a small frying pan, heat oil over medium–high heat. Remove pan from heat and stir in garam masala and chili powder. Pour hot tempering over lentils and stir to mix well.
5. Transfer to a serving dish and top with cilantro. Serve hot.

Serves 4–6 (vegetarian menu) with rice and/or bread, 1 or 2 accompaniments, and 1 other vegetarian main dish
Serves 4–6 (meat menu) with rice and/or bread, 1 or 2 accompaniments, and 1 chicken, meat or seafood main dish
Serves 6–8 (vegetarian menu) with rice and/or bread, 1 or 2 accompaniments, and 2 other vegetarian main dishes
Serves 6–8 (meat menu) with rice and/or bread, 1 or 2 accompaniments, 1 other vegetarian main dish, and 1 chicken, meat or seafood main dish

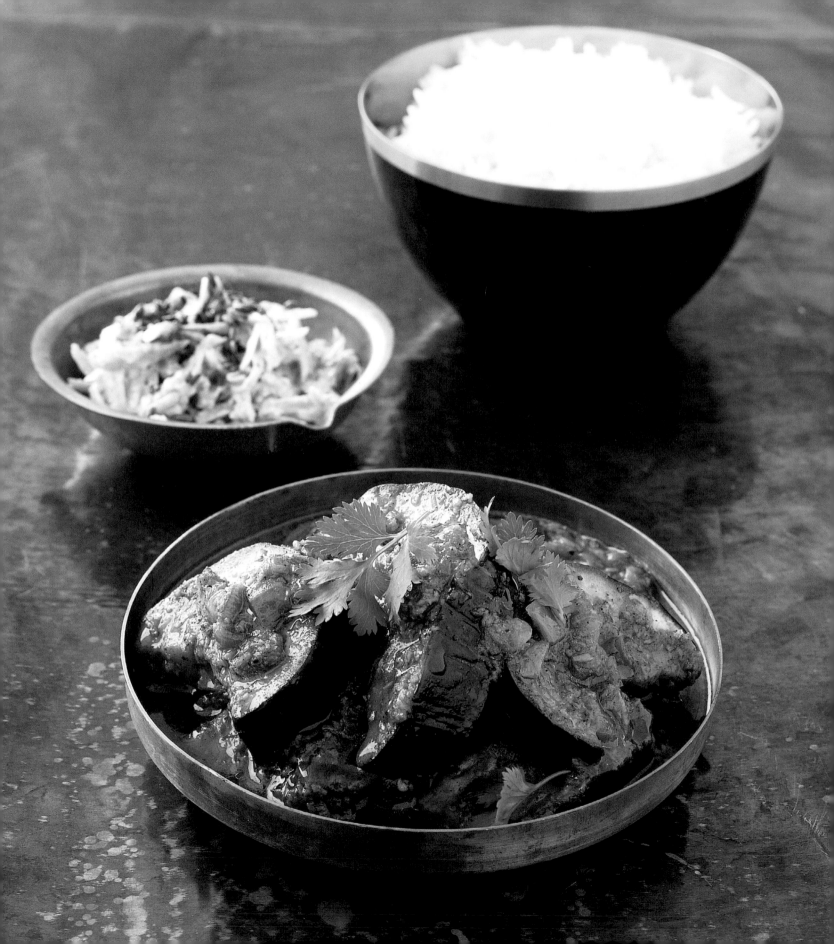

Eggplant with coconut
Masalyachi vangi

1 tablespoon coriander seeds
1 teaspoon black peppercorns
4 whole cloves
¼ cup (1 oz/30 g) desiccated coconut
1 tablespoon minced garlic
½ teaspoon ground turmeric
2 teaspoons salt
**1–2 tablespoons plus ³/₄ cup
(6 fl oz/180 ml) water**
2 tablespoons vegetable oil
2 yellow (brown) onions, finely chopped
**2 eggplants (aubergines), about 12 oz
(375 g) each, halved lengthwise and
cut crosswise into slices ¹/₂ inch
(12 mm) thick**
**Chopped fresh cilantro (fresh
coriander) for garnish**

**Steamed Basmati Rice (page 141)
and/or Home-style Bread (page 141)
for serving
Mango Chutney (page 140) and/or
Carrot and Roast Peanut Relish (page
140) for serving**

This simple, yet refreshing home-style dish comes from the landlords of Marathwada who prepared it on festive occasions.

1. In a small, nonstick pan, combine coriander, peppercorns and cloves over medium heat and dry-roast until fragrant, 2–3 minutes. Let cool slightly, then transfer to a spice grinder and grind to a fine powder. Add coconut to pan and dry-roast over medium heat, stirring, until golden, 2–3 minutes.
2. In a small food processor, combine ground spices, coconut, garlic, turmeric and 1 teaspoon salt. Add just enough water, 1–2 tablespoons, to grind to a smooth paste.
3. In a heavy-bottomed saucepan, heat oil over medium–low heat. Add onions and remaining 1 teaspoon salt and cook uncovered, stirring, until onions are dark golden brown, 20–25 minutes.
4. Raise heat to medium, add spice paste and cook, stirring, for 2 minutes. Add eggplants and ³/₄ cup (6 fl oz/180 ml) water and toss to combine. Reduce heat to medium–low, cover and cook until eggplants are tender, about 20 minutes.
5. Transfer to a serving dish and sprinkle with cilantro. Serve hot.

Serves 4–6 (vegetarian menu) with rice and/or bread, 1 or 2 accompaniments, and Red Lentil Dal (page 137)
Serves 4–6 (meat menu) with rice and/or bread, 1 or 2 accompaniments, and 1 chicken, meat or seafood main dish
Serves 6–8 (vegetarian menu) with rice and/or bread, 1 or 2 accompaniments, Red Lentil Dal (page 137), and 1 other vegetarian main dish
Serves 6–8 (meat menu) with rice and/or bread, 1 or 2 accompaniments, 1 other vegetarian main dish, and 1 chicken, meat or seafood main dish

Eggplant with coconut (front),
carrot and roast peanut relish (back left),
steamed basmati rice (back right)

Accompaniments

Carrot and roast peanut relish
Gajjar chi koshumbiri

10 oz (300 g) carrots, peeled and grated
¹/₂ cup (4 oz/125 g) plain whole-milk
yogurt, whisked until smooth
2 tablespoons unsalted roasted
peanuts, finely chopped
1 fresh mild long green chili,
finely chopped
1 teaspoon sugar
Salt

For Tempering
1 tablespoon vegetable oil
Pinch powdered asafetida
1 teaspoon cumin seeds

Chopped fresh cilantro (fresh
coriander) for garnish

An excellent accompaniment to any meal.

1. In a bowl, combine carrots, yogurt, peanuts, chili and sugar and stir to combine. Season to taste with salt. Transfer to a serving bowl.
2. To make tempering: In a small frying pan, heat oil over medium–high heat. Add asafetida and cumin and cook until seeds start to pop, 1–2 minutes. Remove from heat and pour hot tempering over carrot mixture.
3. Top with cilantro and serve.

Note: This relish tastes best when made just before serving.

Serves 6–8

Mango chutney
Aam ki chatni

1³/₄ cups (14 oz/440 g) sugar
¹/₂ cup (4 fl oz/125 ml) white vinegar
1-inch (2.5-cm) piece fresh ginger,
peeled and cut into thin slices
5 cloves garlic, smashed
2 teaspoons chili powder
1 teaspoon ground turmeric (optional)
1 tablespoon raisins (optional)
1 teaspoon salt
1 lb (500 g) green mangoes, unpeeled,
pitted and grated

An excellent accompaniment to any meal.

1. In a heavy-bottomed saucepan, combine sugar, vinegar, ginger, garlic, chili powder, turmeric and raisins if using, and salt. Stir over low heat until sugar dissolves and mixture is well combined. Bring to a boil and remove from heat. Set aside to cool.
2. Stir in grated mango. Transfer to a jar with a tight-fitting lid. Set aside in a cool, dry place until mango pieces start to soften, at least 4 days.
3. Once opened, refrigerate for up to 2 weeks. Use a clean spoon each time you remove chutney to prevent mold from forming.

Makes about 3 cups

Steamed basmati rice
Sused chawal

2¹/₂ cups (1 lb/500 g) basmati rice
5 cups (40 fl oz/1.25 L) water
¹/₂ teaspoon salt

1. Rinse rice under cold running water until water runs clear. Place rice in a bowl and cover with plenty of cold water. Set aside to soak for 20 minutes.
2. Drain water from rice into a large, heavy saucepan with a tight-fitting lid. Add salt and bring to a boil over medium–high heat. Add soaked rice, stir once and then bring to a boil. Reduce heat to low, cover partially and cook until most of the water is absorbed and steam holes appear in the surface of rice, 10–15 minutes.
3. Remove from heat and set aside for 5 minutes without lifting lid.
4. Fluff grains with a fork and serve.

Serves 8–10

Note: You can easily halve or double this recipe.

Home-style bread
Phulka

2 cups (10 oz/300 g) whole-wheat
(wholemeal) flour
1 teaspoon salt
²/₃ cup (5 fl oz/150 ml) plus
1 tablespoon water
Melted unsalted butter

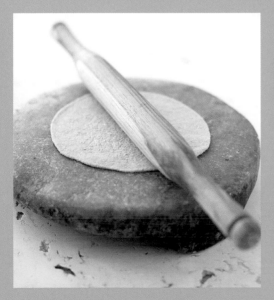

1. In a large bowl, stir together flour and salt. Make a well in center. Gradually add ²/₃ cup (5 fl oz/150 ml) water in small amounts to center and, using your hand, work into dry ingredients until a soft dough forms. Turn out onto a lightly floured surface and knead until very smooth, about 15 minutes. Place dough in a lightly oiled bowl and sprinkle with 1 tablespoon water. Cover bowl with a clean, damp kitchen towel and set aside for 20 minutes.
2. Turn out dough again onto lightly floured surface and knead for a further 5–10 minutes. Dough should be smooth.
3. Divide dough into 12 equal portions. Shape each portion into a ball, and then roll out each ball into a disk about 5 inches (13 cm) in diameter.
4. Heat a heavy cast-iron griddle or a grill pan over medium heat. When hot, place a disk of dough on griddle and cook, lightly pressing disk all over with a clean, dry kitchen towel (use a dabbing motion), until disk is golden brown in spots on underside, 1–2 minutes. Turn and cook on second side until golden brown in spots and cooked through, about 1 minute longer.
5. Remove griddle from heat. If you have a gas stove, you can hold the bread over the open flame until it puffs up, 10–20 seconds. If you have an electric stove, omit this step. Set bread aside and keep hot. Cook remaining breads in same way.
6. Brush 1 side of bread with butter and transfer to a serving tray. Repeat with remaining breads. Serve hot.

Makes 12

Desserts

Stuffed bananas
Bhareli keli

3 tablespoons unsalted butter
3½ oz (100 g) jaggery, grated
2 teaspoons ground green cardamom pods (ground in spice grinder)
½ cup (2 oz/60 g) desiccated coconut
6 small ripe bananas
1 can (13 fl oz/400 ml) coconut milk

1. In a large nonstick frying pan, combine butter, jaggery and cardamom. Place over low heat until butter and jaggery melt. Raise heat to medium and add coconut. Cook, stirring, for 3 minutes. Remove pan from heat and set aside to cool.
2. Peel bananas and cut in half lengthwise, stopping about 3/4 inch (2 cm) short of opposite end. Carefully stuff coconut mixture into middle of bananas.
3. Place bananas in pan with butter and jaggery and pour over coconut milk. Place over medium heat and bring to a simmer. Cook, uncovered, until bananas are soft but still hold their shape, 10–15 minutes.
4. Transfer to individual plates and top with sauce. Serve warm.

Serves 6

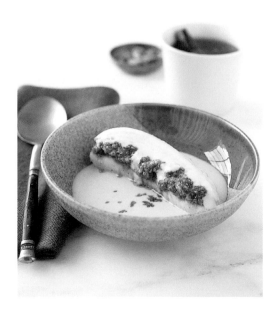

Saffron-flavored sweetened yogurt
Shrikhand

4 cups (2 lb/1 kg) plain whole-milk yogurt
¹/₂ teaspoon saffron threads, soaked in ¹/₃ cup (3 fl oz/90 ml) warm whole milk for 10 minutes
¹/₃ cup (2¹/₂ oz/75 g) superfine (caster) sugar, plus more to taste if needed
¹/₄–¹/₂ teaspoon ground green cardamom pods (ground in spice grinder)
1 tablespoon almond meal
Slivered blanched almonds for garnish

This pale-hued yogurt is a favorite dessert not only in Maharashtra, but across India.

1. Line a sieve with a double layer of damp cheesecloth (muslin) and place over bowl. Pour in yogurt and cover sieve. Refrigerate until most of liquid, or whey, has drained out of yogurt, about 2 hours.
2. Pour yogurt from sieve into a bowl. Stir in saffron and milk and ¹/₃ cup (2¹/₂ oz/75 g) sugar. Mix well. Stir in ¹/₄ teaspoon cardamom and almond meal. Taste and adjust with sugar and cardamom if necessary. Cover and refrigerate for 2 hours to allow flavors to develop.
3. Divide yogurt among individual bowls. Top with slivered almonds and serve.

Serves 6

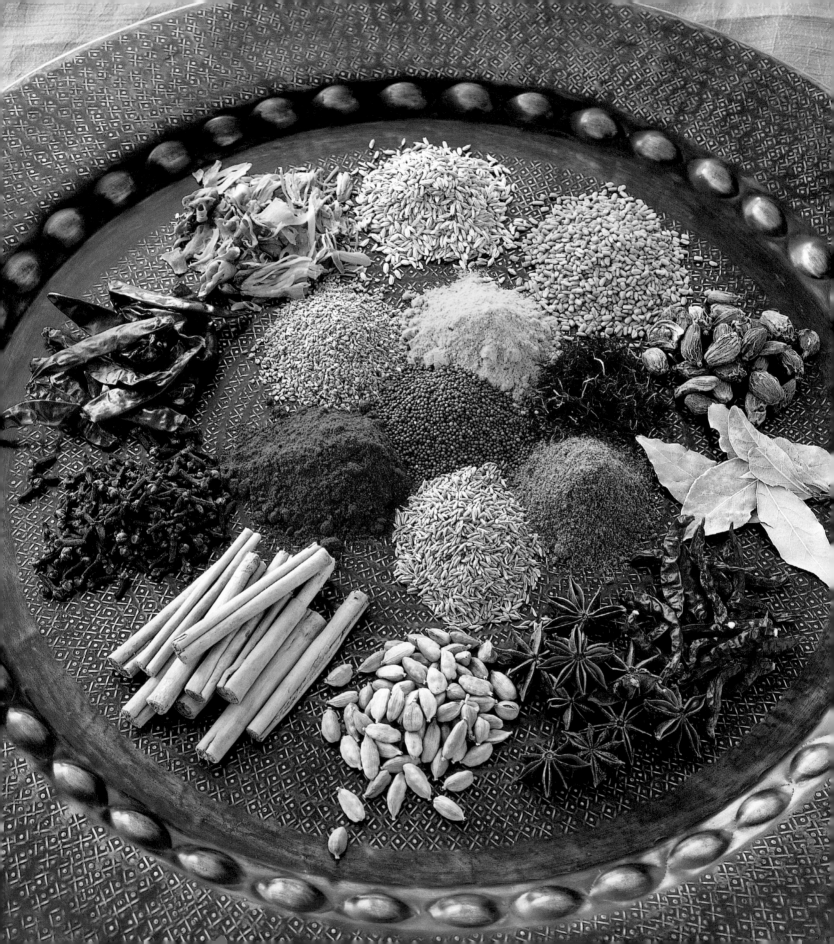

Central India

Introduction

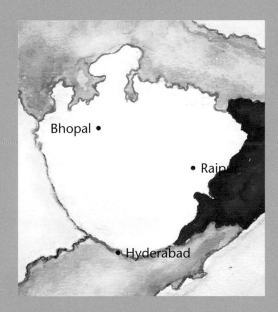

The Central Region of India, or Deccan, is the place to which I belong and is home to some 80-100 million people. The state of Madhya Pradesh is considered to be the center of India and the region also consists of some parts of Andhra Pradesh, Karnataka and Maharashtra.

This is the hottest region in the country with temperatures ranging from 95–105°F (35–40°C), although some parts of Maharashtra, south of its capital Mumbai, can experience heavy rainfalls. Maharashtra, which is also renowned for its sophisticated lifestyle and industrialization, is situated in west-central India. Mumbai is considered the business capital of India and is home to the famous "Bollywood," which is the center of India's film industry.

Karnataka, which is south of Andra Pradesh, is also considered to be part of the southern region of India. Bangalore, which is where I became an executive chef with the Taj Group, is the capital of Karnataka. The Usha restaurant, where I received much inspiration, is in Mangalore, which is one of the other major cities of Karnataka.

The main produce of the Central Region includes sugar, hot varieties of chili, and turmeric, which is stored in vast deep pits in the ground. This region is also famous for its mangoes, like Jehangir, Begunpalli and Be-Nishan, and custard apples.

To me, the food from this region comes as close as any to defining Indian food – if there is such a thing. This region has taken the best of the North, East, West and South regions and some of the overseas influences that India has absorbed over the past thousand years or more, and has combined all these flavors to create a unique, subtle cuisine.

Most dishes from this region are meat based. However, the regional dishes also make use of lentils and vegetables, such as the Dalcha Gosht, which is a combination of lamb and lentils. This region is home to the famous Hyderabadi Biriyani and Dum ke Kebab.

Food from this region of India is rich but highly digestible, hot yet mild on the palate. Best of all, the food of the Central Region is extremely easy to prepare. This is because it uses two of the most important ingredients for cooking – fursat (leisure) and mohabbat (love).

Enjoy the spicy yet flavorsome cuisine of Central Indian food!

Starters

Dry-roasted lamb
Sukka lamb

1 lb (500 g) boneless lamb shoulder (blade), cut into 1-inch (2.5-cm) pieces
2 teaspoons minced garlic
2 teaspoons grated fresh ginger
2 cups (16 fl oz/500 ml) water
1¹/2 teaspoons salt
¹/2 teaspoon ground turmeric
5 tablespoons vegetable oil
2 yellow (brown) onions, halved and thinly sliced
¹/3 cup (1¹/2 oz/45 g) desiccated coconut
2 teaspoons coriander seeds
1 teaspoon cumin seeds
2-inch (5-cm) piece cinnamon stick
4 whole cloves
2 green cardamom pods
1 teaspoon chili powder
Leaves from 1 bunch fresh cilantro (fresh coriander), chopped
Juice of 1 lime

This Dakhni lamb is extremely popular with the Muslims of Hyderabad.

1. In a bowl, combine lamb, garlic and ginger and toss to coat lamb evenly. Set aside for 10 minutes.
2. In a saucepan, combine lamb mixture, water and ¹/2 teaspoon salt. Bring to a simmer over medium heat, cover partially and simmer until lamb is very tender, 45–60 minutes. Drain off any excess liquid.
3. Meanwhile, in a frying pan, heat 2 tablespoons oil over medium–low heat. Add onions and remaining 1 teaspoon salt and cook uncovered, stirring occasionally, until onions are dark golden brown, 20–25 minutes. Remove from pan and set aside.
4. In a spice grinder, combine coconut, coriander, cumin, cinnamon, cloves and cardamom and grind to a fine powder.
5. In a frying pan, heat remaining 3 tablespoons oil over high heat. Add lamb and cook, stirring and tossing, until well browned, 3–4 minutes. Stir in ground spice mix and chili powder. Cook, stirring and tossing, until fragrant, 2–3 minutes.
6. Taste and adjust seasoning with salt if necessary. Add fried onions, cilantro and lime juice to lamb and toss well. Transfer to a serving plate and serve hot.

Serves 4 as starter
Serves 6–8 as starter with 1 other starter
Serves 8–10 as starter with all 3 starters

Dry roasted lamb (front),
home-style chicken kebabs (back)

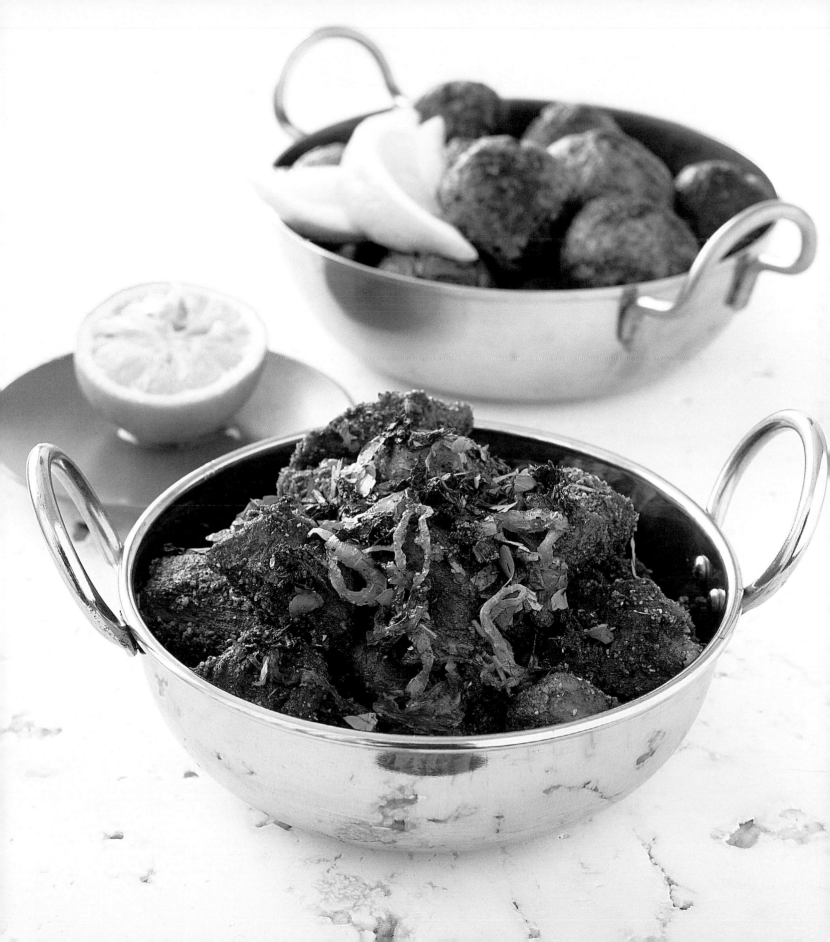

Home-style chicken kebabs
Dum ke kebab

1 teaspoon plus 2 tablespoons vegetable oil, plus oil for brushing grill pan
2-inch (5-cm) piece cinnamon stick
2 yellow (brown) onions, halved and thinly sliced
1 teaspoon salt
1 lb (500 g) ground (minced) chicken
Leaves from 1/2 bunch fresh mint, chopped
Leaves from 1/2 bunch fresh cilantro (fresh coriander), chopped
1 teaspoon minced garlic
1 teaspoon grated fresh ginger
1 teaspoon Nilgiri's Garam Masala (page 28)
Lemon wedges for serving

This is the Nizami version of the Mogul Royalty's "nabob kebab."

1. In a small, nonstick frying pan, heat 1 teaspoon oil over medium heat. Add cinnamon and cook until dark golden brown, 3–4 minutes. Set aside to cool completely, and then grind in a spice grinder to a fine powder.
2. In a frying pan, heat 2 tablespoons oil over medium–low heat. Add onions and salt and cook uncovered, stirring occasionally, until onions are dark golden brown, 20–25 minutes. Set aside to cool.
3. In a food processor, combine chicken, mint, cilantro, garlic, ginger, garam masala and fried onions and process until well combined. Use wet hands to shape tablespoonfuls of mixture into balls.
4. Preheat a grill pan over medium heat. Brush with oil. Add meatballs to grill pan and cook, turning often, until well browned, 3–4 minutes. Reduce heat to medium–low, cover and cook until meatballs are cooked through, 8–10 minutes.
5. Arrange meatballs on a serving plate and sprinkle with ground cinnamon. Serve hot with lemon wedges.

Serves 4 as starter
Serves 6–8 as starter with 1 other starter
Serves 8–10 as starter with all 3 starters

Panfried marinated fish
Thali macchi

1 lb (500 g) white fish fillets such as snapper or cod, cut into 1-inch (2.5-cm) thick slices
2 teaspoons coriander seeds, ground in spice grinder
1 teaspoon chili powder
1/2 teaspoon ground turmeric
2 teaspoons minced garlic
1/4 cup (2 fl oz/60 ml) vegetable oil
2 yellow (brown) onions, halved and thinly sliced
1 teaspoon salt

This fried fish brings back memories of the Banjara Hotel in Hyderabad where this was a favorite of the waiting staff whenever they were lucky enough to have it!

1. In a bowl, combine fish, coriander, chili, turmeric and garlic and stir well to coat fish evenly. Set aside for 10 minutes.
2. In a frying pan, heat oil over medium–low heat. Add onions and salt and cook uncovered, stirring occasionally, until onions are dark golden brown, 20–25 minutes. Using a slotted spoon, remove from pan and set aside.
3. Reheat oil over high heat. Working in batches, add fish and cook, turning once, until cooked and golden, 3–4 minutes. As each batch is ready, transfer to a plate.
4. Top fish with caramelized onions and serve hot.

Serves 4 as starter
Serves 6–8 as starter with 1 other starter
Serves 8–10 as starter with all 3 starters

Main Dishes

Hyderabadi-style chicken korma with saffron
Murgh nawabi

1 whole chicken, 3 lb (1.5 kg), cut into 10 pieces, or 2 lb (1 kg) chicken pieces
2 teaspoons minced garlic
2 teaspoons grated fresh ginger
¹/₄ cup (2 oz/60 g) plain whole-milk yogurt
2 teaspoons salt
2 dried red chilies
2 teaspoons aniseed
¹/₂ cup (4 fl oz/125 ml) vegetable oil
2 yellow (brown) onions, finely chopped
1¹/₂ teaspoons Nilgiri's Garam Masala (page 28)
¹/₂ cup (4 fl oz/125 ml) water
¹/₂ teaspoon saffron threads, soaked in ¹/₂ cup (4 fl oz/125 ml) warm whole milk for 10 minutes
3 eggs, hard-boiled and peeled
¹/₄ cup (1¹/₂ oz/45 g) raisins
¹/₄ cup (1¹/₂ oz/45 g) raw cashew nuts (optional)

Steamed Basmati Rice (page 141) and/or Home-style Bread (page 141) for serving
Onion Raita (page 168), Sesame Seed Chutney (page 168), Tomato Pickle (page 169) and/or Garlic and Red Chili Chutney (page 169) for serving

This is the best Korma recipe in the world!

1. In a bowl, combine chicken, garlic, ginger, yogurt and 1 teaspoon salt and mix until well combined. Set aside.
2. In a spice grinder, combine chilies and aniseed and grind to a fine powder. Set aside.
3. In a heavy-bottomed saucepan, heat ¹/₄ cup (2 fl oz/60 ml) oil over medium–low heat. Add onions and remaining 1 teaspoon salt and cook uncovered, stirring occasionally, until onions are softened, 10–15 minutes. Stir in ground spices and garam masala and cook, stirring, until fragrant, 2–3 minutes.
4. Raise heat to high, add chicken and cook, turning occasionally, until browned, 4–5 minutes. Stir in water, reduce heat to medium–low, cover partially and cook until chicken is cooked through and tender, about 20 minutes. Remove pan from heat and stir in saffron and milk. Set aside.
5. In a small, nonstick frying pan, heat remaining ¹/₄ cup (2 fl oz/60 ml) oil over medium–high heat. Add eggs and cook, turning often, until golden brown, 2–3 minutes. Using a slotted spoon, transfer to a plate lined with paper towels to drain. Reduce heat to medium, add raisins and cashew nuts if using, and cook, tossing, until golden, 1–2 minutes. Using a slotted spoon, transfer to paper towels to drain.
6. Arrange chicken on a serving plate and top with eggs, raisins and cashew nuts. Serve immediately.

Serves 4–6 with rice and/or bread and 1 or more accompaniments
Serves 6–8 with rice and/or bread, 1 or more accompaniments, 1 vegetarian main dish, and 1 meat or seafood main dish

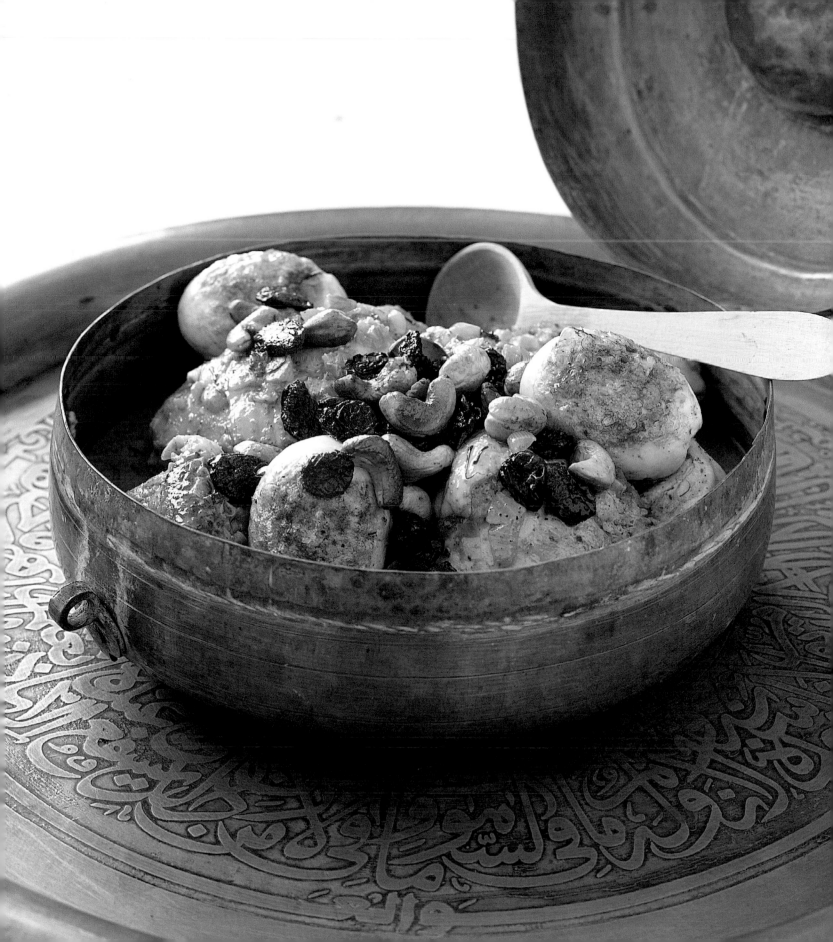

Chicken khurma with tomatoes and coconut
Hyderabadi khurma

6 tablespoons vegetable oil
3 yellow (brown) onions, halved and thinly sliced
1 teaspoon salt
8 whole blanched almonds (optional)
6 whole unsalted roasted cashew nuts (optional)
4 whole cloves
2-inch (5-cm) piece cinnamon stick, broken into small pieces
3 green cardamom pods
1/4 cup (1 oz/30 g) desiccated coconut
2 or 3 dried red chilies, broken into small pieces
1 tablespoon minced garlic
2 teaspoons grated fresh ginger
2 large, ripe tomatoes, chopped
3 lb (1.5 kg) whole chicken, cut into 10 pieces or 2 lb (1 kg) chicken pieces
1 cup (8 fl oz/250 ml) water
1/2 teaspoon saffron threads, soaked in 1/2 cup (4 fl oz/125 ml) warm whole milk
2 tablespoons powdered whole milk

Steamed Basmati Rice (page 141) and/or Home-style Bread (page 141) for serving
Onion Raita (page 168), Sesame Seed Chutney (page 168), Tomato Pickle (page 169) and/or Garlic and Red Chili Chutney (page 169) for serving

Second only to the Murgh Nawabi Korma, this khurma uses tomatoes and coconut.

1. In a heavy-bottomed saucepan, heat 2 tablespoons oil over medium–low heat. Add onions and salt and cook uncovered, stirring occasionally, until onions are dark golden brown, 20–25 minutes. Remove from pan.
2. Meanwhile, in a spice grinder, combine almonds and cashew nuts if using, cloves, cinnamon, cardamom, coconut and chilies and grind finely.
3. Heat remaining 4 tablespoons oil in saucepan over medium heat. Add ground spices and cook, stirring, until fragrant, 2–3 minutes. Stir in garlic, ginger and tomatoes and cook, stirring, for about 5 minutes. Raise heat to high, add chicken and cook, turning occasionally, until browned, 4–5 minutes.
4. Stir fried onions and water into pan. Reduce heat to medium–low, cover partially and simmer for 10 minutes. Stir in saffron and milk and milk powder and continue to simmer, uncovered, until chicken is cooked through and tender, 10–15 minutes longer.
5. Taste and adjust seasoning with salt if necessary. Transfer to a serving dish and serve hot.

Serves 4–6 with rice and/or bread and 1 or more accompaniments
Serves 6–8 with rice and/or bread, 1 or more accompaniments, 1 vegetarian main dish, and 1 meat or seafood main dish

Note: The difference between a khurma and a korma is the latter dish does not contain coconut.

Chicken in green herbs

Hare masale ki murgi

5 tablespoons vegetable oil
3 yellow (brown) onions, halved and thinly sliced
1 teaspoon salt
1 whole chicken, 3 lb (1.5 kg), cut into 10 pieces, or 2 lb (1 kg) chicken pieces
1/2 cup (4 oz/125 g) plain whole-milk yogurt, whisked until smooth
1 tablespoon grated fresh ginger
1 tablespoon minced garlic
2-inch (5-cm) piece cinnamon stick, broken into small pieces
8 whole black peppercorns
4 green cardamom pods
2 teaspoons coriander seeds
1 teaspoon cumin seeds
4 fresh mild long green chilies, roughly chopped
Leaves from 1 bunch fresh cilantro (fresh coriander)
Leaves from 1 bunch fresh mint
1 tablespoon unsalted roasted cashew nuts (optional)
1/4 teaspoon ground turmeric
1/2 cup (4 fl oz/125 ml) water
2 tablespoons heavy (double) cream

Steamed Basmati Rice (page 141) and/or Home-style Bread (page 141) for serving
Onion Raita (page 168), Sesame Seed Chutney (page 168), Tomato Pickle (page 169) and/or Garlic and Red Chili Chutney (page 169) for serving

This home-style dish is not only popular in every household in Hyderabad but also in the city's restaurants.

1. In a frying pan, heat 2 tablespoons oil over medium–low heat. Add onions and salt and cook, stirring occasionally, until onions are dark golden brown, 20–25 minutes. Using a slotted spoon, transfer onions to a plate.
2. Meanwhile, in a bowl, combine chicken, yogurt, ginger and garlic and stir to coat chicken evenly. Set aside.
3. In a spice grinder, combine cinnamon, peppercorns, cardamom, coriander and cumin and grind to a fine powder. In a small food processor, combine chilies, cilantro, mint, cashew nuts if using, and fried onions. Process until well combined.
4. In a frying pan, heat remaining 3 tablespoons oil over high heat. Add chicken and cook, turning occasionally, until all moisture evaporates and chicken is lightly browned, 4–5 minutes. Stir turmeric and water into pan, reduce heat to medium–low heat, cover partially and cook until chicken is cooked through and tender, 20–25 minutes.
5. Add ground spices and cook, stirring, until fragrant, 2–3 minutes. Stir in cilantro mixture and cream and cook, stirring, until mixture is well combined and heated through, 3–4 minutes.
6. Taste and adjust seasoning with salt if necessary. Transfer to a serving dish and serve hot.

Serves 4–6 with rice and/or bread and 1 or more accompaniments
Serves 6–8 with rice and/or bread, 1 or more accompaniments, 1 vegetarian main dish, and 1 meat or seafood main dish

Home-style meat broth
Lamb shorva

¹/₃ cup (3 fl oz/90 ml) vegetable oil
5 yellow (brown) onions, chopped
1 teaspoon salt
5 green cardamom pods
5 whole cloves
2 bay leaves
2-inch (5-cm) piece cinnamon stick
1 tablespoon coriander seeds,
ground in spice grinder
1 teaspoon ground turmeric
1 tablespoon minced garlic
2 teaspoons grated fresh ginger
1¹/₂ lb (750 g) boneless lamb shoulder
(blade), cut into 1-inch (2.5-cm) pieces
4 fresh mild long green chilies,
slit lengthwise
4 ripe tomatoes, chopped
1 cup (8 fl oz/250 ml) vegetable stock
1 teaspoon Nilgiri's Garam Masala
(page 28)
Leaves from 1 bunch fresh cilantro
(fresh coriander), chopped
2 eggs, hard-boiled, peeled and
quartered (optional)

Steamed Basmati Rice (page 141)
and/or Home-style Bread (page 141)
for serving
Onion Raita (page 168), Sesame Seed
Chutney (page 168), Tomato Pickle
(page 169) and/or Garlic and Red Chili
Chutney (page 169) for serving

This nutritious, filling and tasty dish is normally eaten by Muslims during Ramzan.

1. In a large, heavy-bottomed saucepan, heat oil over medium–low heat. Add onions and salt and cook uncovered, stirring often, until onions are softened, 10–15 minutes.
2. Raise heat to medium and stir in cardamom, cloves, bay leaves, cinnamon, coriander and turmeric. Cook, stirring, until fragrant, 2–3 minutes. Stir in garlic and ginger and cook, stirring, for 1 minute. Raise heat to high, add lamb and cook until browned, 3–4 minutes.
3. Add chilies, tomatoes and stock to pan, cover partially and cook, stirring occasionally, until meat is very tender, 45–60 minutes.
4. Taste and adjust seasoning with salt if necessary. Transfer to a serving dish and sprinkle with garam masala, cilantro and eggs if using. Serve hot.

Serves 4–6 with rice and/or bread and 1 or more accompaniments
Serves 6–8 with rice and/or bread, 1 or more accompaniments, 1 vegetarian main dish, and 1 chicken or seafood main dish

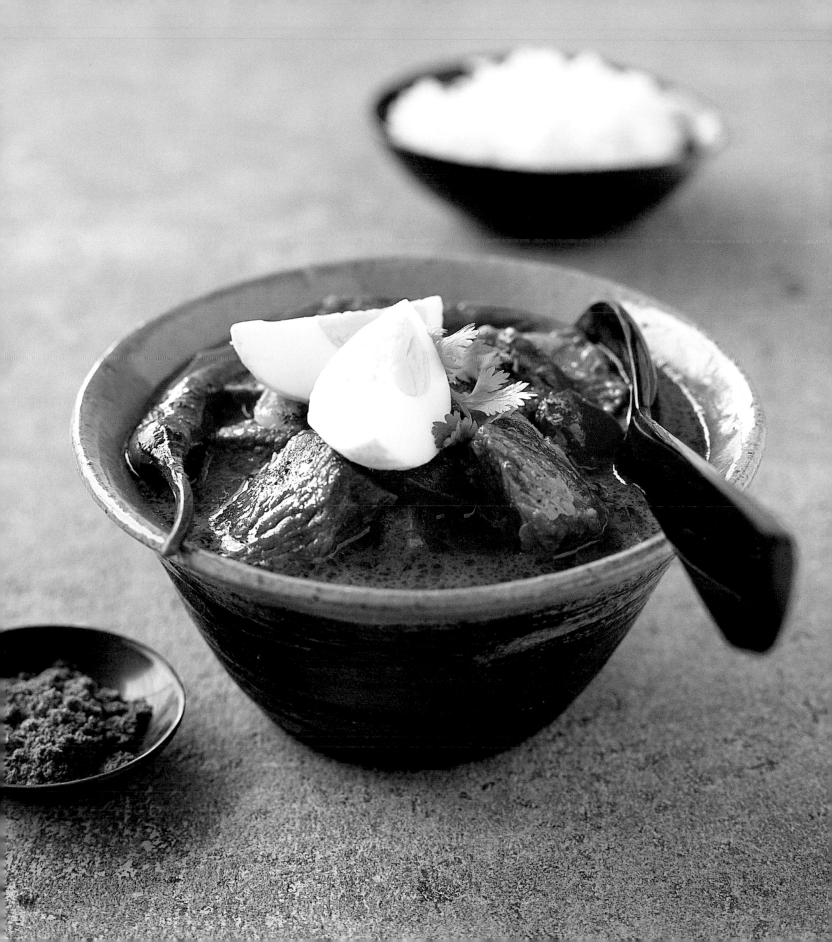

Lamb kebabs
Kacche kebab

1 yellow (brown) onion, roughly chopped
4 fresh mild long green chilies, roughly chopped
Leaves from 1 bunch fresh mint, roughly chopped
1 teaspoon minced garlic
1 teaspoon grated fresh ginger
1 teaspoon coriander seeds
1 teaspoon cumin seeds
1 lb (500 g) ground (minced) lamb
1 teaspoon Nilgiri's Garam Masala (page 28)
1 teaspoon chili powder (optional)
1 teaspoon salt
1 small egg, whisked until blended
2 tablespoons vegetable oil

Steamed Basmati Rice (page 141) and/or Home-style Bread (page 141) for serving

Onion Raita (page 168), Sesame Seed Chutney (page 168), Tomato Pickle (page 169) and/or Garlic and Red Chili Chutney (page 169) for serving

This is an excellent, easy-to-make dish for any household.

1. In a small food processor, combine onion, chilies, mint, garlic and ginger and process until finely chopped and well combined. In a spice grinder, combine coriander and cumin seeds and grind to a fine powder.
2. In a bowl, combine lamb, garam masala, chili powder if using, salt, onion mixture and ground spices. Use your hands to mix until well combined. Add egg and again mix until well combined. Moisten hands with water, divide mixture into 12 equal portions, and then shape each portion into a round patty. Cover and refrigerate for 30 minutes.
3. In a large, heavy-bottomed nonstick frying pan, heat oil over medium heat. Working in batches if necessary, add patties and fry, turning once, until cooked through, 3–4 minutes on each side.
4. Transfer to a serving plate and serve hot.

Serves 4–6 with rice and/or bread and 1 or more accompaniments
Serves 6–8 with rice and/or bread, 1 or more accompaniments, 1 vegetarian main dish, and 1 chicken or seafood main dish

Lamb and chickpeas
Dalcha

3/4 cup (5 oz/150 g) split chickpea lentils
1/3 cup (3 fl oz/90 ml) vegetable oil
4 yellow (brown) onions, halved and thinly sliced
1 teaspoon salt
1 lb (500 g) lamb shoulder (blade), cut into 1-inch (2.5-cm) pieces
2 teaspoons minced garlic
2 teaspoons grated fresh ginger
1¹/₂ teaspoons coriander seeds, ground in spice grinder
1 teaspoon chili powder
¹/₂ teaspoon ground turmeric
3 cups (24 fl oz/750 ml) water
4 fresh mild long green chilies, slit lengthwise
Juice of 1 lime

Steamed Basmati Rice (page 141) and/or Home-style Bread (page 141) for serving
Onion Raita (page 168), Sesame Seed Chutney (page 168), Tomato Pickle (page 169) and/or Garlic and Red Chili Chutney (page 169) for serving

A potpourri of lamb and chickpeas cooked to perfection.

1. Rinse chickpea lentils. In a bowl, combine chickpea lentils with plenty of cold water to cover. Set aside for 30 minutes to soak. Drain, then rinse and drain well. Set aside.
2. Meanwhile, in a large frying pan, heat oil over medium–low heat. Add onions and salt and cook uncovered, stirring occasionally, until onions are dark golden brown, 20–25 minutes. Transfer half of fried onions to a plate lined with paper towels and set aside.
3. Raise heat to high and add lamb to onions remaining in pan. Cook, stirring and tossing, until meat is browned, 2–3 minutes. Add garlic, ginger, coriander, chili powder and turmeric and cook, stirring, until fragrant, 2–3 minutes.
4. Add chickpea lentils and water to pan and stir to combine. Reduce heat to medium–low, cover partially and simmer until meat is very tender and lentils break down to form a rich sauce, 45–60 minutes.
5. Remove pan from heat. Stir chilies and lime juice into pan and then taste and adjust seasoning with salt. Transfer to a serving dish and top with reserved fried onions. Serve hot.

Serves 4–6 with rice and/or bread and 1 or more accompaniments
Serves 6–8 with rice and/or bread, 1 or more accompaniments, 1 vegetarian main dish, and 1 chicken or seafood main dish

Seafood Recipes

Hyderabadi-style fish stew
Macchi ka salan

3 tablespoons vegetable oil
2 brown (yellow) onions, halved and
thinly sliced, plus 1 onion, chopped
1 teaspoon salt
2 teaspoons sesame seeds
2 teaspoons coriander seeds
1 teaspoon cumin seeds
1 teaspoon black or brown
mustard seeds
1 cup (4 oz/125 g) desiccated coconut
2 teaspoons chili powder
¹/2 teaspoon ground turmeric
2 teaspoons minced garlic
1¹/2 lb (750 g) white fish fillets such
as snapper or cod, cut into slices
1 inch (2.5 cm) thick
1 can (13 fl oz/400 ml) coconut milk
20 fresh curry leaves
2 fresh mild long green chilies,
slit lengthwise
1 teaspoon tamarind concentrate
2 tablespoons chopped fresh cilantro
(fresh coriander)

Steamed Basmati Rice (page 141)
and/or Home-style Bread (page 141)
for serving
Onion Raita (page 168), Sesame Seed
Chutney (page 168), Tomato Pickle
(page 169) and/or Garlic and Red Chili
Chutney (page 169) for serving

After biryani, the preparation of this dish is the ultimate test of a Hyderabadi chef.

1. In a large frying pan, heat oil over medium–low heat. Add sliced onions and salt and cook uncovered, stirring occasionally, until onions are dark golden brown, 20–25 minutes.
2. Meanwhile, in a spice grinder, combine sesame, coriander, cumin and mustard seeds and grind to a fine powder. Transfer ground spices to a small food processor and add coconut, chili powder, turmeric, garlic and chopped onion. Process until well combined.
3. When onions are ready, raise heat to medium, add spice mixture and cook, stirring, until fragrant, 3–4 minutes. Add fish, coconut milk, curry leaves, chilies and tamarind. Stir to combine and simmer, uncovered, until fish is just cooked and flakes when tested with a fork, 10–15 minutes.
4. Taste and adjust seasoning with salt if necessary. Transfer to a serving dish and top with cilantro. Serve hot.

Serves 4–6 with rice and/or bread and 1 or more accompaniments
Serves 6–8 with rice and/or bread, 1 or more accompaniments, 1 vegetarian main dish, and 1 chicken or lamb main dish

Hyderabadi-style fish stew (center),
tomato pickle (left)

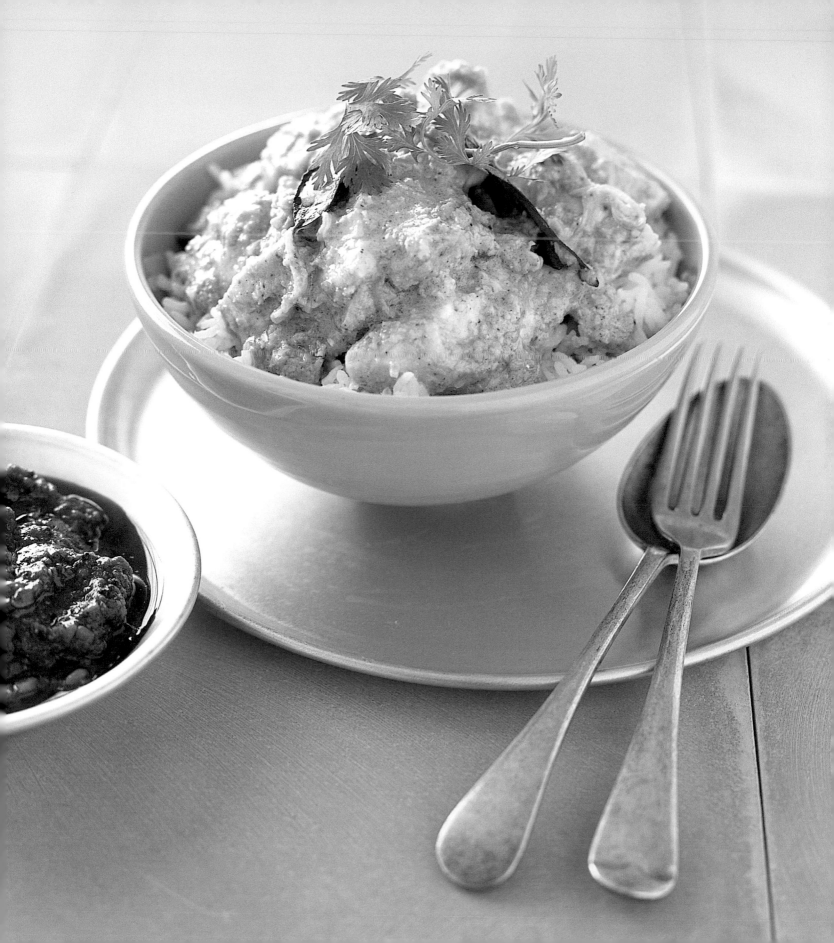

Sweet-and-sour fish
Khatti machali

1¹/₂ lb (750 g) white fish fillets such as snapper or cod, cut into slices 1 inch (2.5 cm) thick
2 teaspoons minced garlic
2 teaspoons grated fresh ginger
1–2 teaspoons chili powder
¹/₂ teaspoon ground turmeric
1 teaspoon salt
4 large, ripe tomatoes, about 12 oz (375 g) total weight
3 tablespoons vegetable oil
¹/₂ teaspoon fenugreek seeds
1 cup (8 fl oz/250 ml) water
20 fresh curry leaves
1 teaspoon tamarind concentrate
¹/₄ cup (¹/₃ oz/10 g) chopped fresh cilantro (fresh coriander)

Steamed Basmati Rice (page 141) and/or Home-style Bread (page 141) for serving
Onion Raita (page 168), Sesame Seed Chutney (page 168), Tomato Pickle (page 169) and/or Garlic and Red Chili Chutney (page 169) for serving

This is a Hyderabadi version of the Andhra Pradesh classic.

1. In a bowl, combine fish, garlic, ginger, chili powder (use larger amount if you want more heat), turmeric and salt and toss to coat fish evenly. Set aside.
2. Using a small knife, remove core from each tomato. Make a small, shallow cross in blossom end (bottom) of each tomato. Place in a large heatproof bowl and cover with plenty of boiling water. Set aside for 10 minutes. Drain and peel away skin. Place tomatoes in a food processor and process until pureed.
3. In a frying pan, heat oil over medium heat. Add fenugreek and cook, stirring, for 2–3 minutes. Carefully stir in tomato puree and water and simmer, uncovered, for about 10 minutes.
4. Add fish, curry leaves and tamarind to pan and stir well. Continue to simmer, uncovered, over medium heat until fish is just cooked and flakes when tested with a fork, 10–15 minutes.
5. Taste and adjust seasoning with salt if necessary. Transfer to a serving dish and top with cilantro or stir cilantro in mixture. Serve hot.

Serves 4–6 with rice and/or bread and 1 or more accompaniments
Serves 6–8 with rice and/or bread, 1 or more accompaniments, 1 vegetarian main dish, and 1 chicken or meat main dish

Shrimp pulao, Deccan style

Jingha pullao

2¹/₂ cups (1 lb/500 g) basmati rice
1 yellow (brown) onion,
roughly chopped
¹/₂ cup (¹/₂oz/15 q) fresh mint leaves
2 teaspoons poppy seeds (optional)
4 fresh mild long green chilies,
roughly chopped
1 teaspoon ground turmeric
1 teaspoon minced garlic
1 teaspoon grated fresh ginger
2 lb (1 kg) medium shrimp (prawns),
peeled and deveined
¹/₃ cup (3 fl oz/90 ml) vegetable oil
2-inch (5-cm) piece cinnamon stick
4 whole cloves
1 bay leaf
3 green cardamom pods
3³/₄ cups (30 fl oz/900 ml) vegetable
stock or water
1 teaspoon salt
1 teaspoon Nilgiri's Garam Masala
(page 28)
¹/₂ cup (³/₄ oz/20 g) chopped fresh
cilantro (fresh coriander)

Home-style Bread (page 141)
Onion Raita (page 168), Sesame Seed
Chutney (page 168), Tomato Pickle
(page 169) and/or Garlic and Red Chili
Chutney (page 169) for serving

1. Rinse rice under cold running water until water runs clear. Place in a bowl and cover with plenty of cold water. Set aside for 20 minutes and then drain well.
2. In a food processor, combine onion, mint, poppy seeds if using, chilies and turmeric and process to a fine paste. Transfer to a bowl and stir in garlic, ginger and shrimp. Set aside for 10 minutes.
3. In a large heavy-bottomed saucepan, heat oil over medium heat. Add marinated shrimp and cook until oil separates, 2–3 minutes. Add cinnamon, cloves, bay leaf, cardamom and drained rice and cook, stirring, for 2 minutes.
4. Pour stock or water into pan and add salt and garam masala. Bring to a simmer, reduce heat to low, cover and cook for 12 minutes. Remove from heat and set aside, covered, until all liquid is absorbed and rice is light and fluffy, 6–8 minutes.
5. Taste and adjust seasoning with salt if necessary. Transfer to a serving dish and top with cilantro. Serve immediately.

Serves 4–6 with bread and 1 or more accompaniments
Serves 6–8 with bread, 1 or more accompaniments, 1 vegetarian main dish, and 1 chicken or meat main dish

Rich tomatoes with cashew nuts
Malai korma

2 tablespoons vegetable oil
2 yellow (brown) onions, chopped
1 teaspoon salt
1 teaspoon minced garlic
1 teaspoon grated fresh ginger
1/2 teaspoon ground turmeric
4 fresh mild long green chilies,
slit lengthwise
3 lb (1.5 kg) ripe tomatoes, chopped
1¹/2 cups (12 fl oz/375 ml) heavy
(double) cream
Leaves from 1 bunch fresh cilantro
(fresh coriander), chopped
2 tablespoons unsalted roasted
cashew nuts, chopped

Steamed Basmati Rice (page 141) or
Coconut Rice (page 85) and/or
Home-style Bread (page 141)
for serving
Onion Raita (page 168), Sesame Seed
Chutney (page 168), Tomato Pickle
(page 169) and/or Garlic and Red Chili
Chutney (page 169) for serving

1. In a heavy-bottomed saucepan, heat oil over medium–low heat. Add onions and salt and cook uncovered, stirring occasionally, until onions are softened, 10–15 minutes. Stir in garlic, ginger, turmeric and chilies and cook, stirring, for 2 minutes.
2. Add tomatoes to pan, raise heat to medium, bring to a simmer and simmer uncovered, stirring occasionally, until tomatoes break down, about 20 minutes.
3. Stir in cream, reduce heat to low and continue to cook, stirring occasionally, until mixture is thick and rich, about 1 hour.
4. Taste and adjust seasoning with salt if necessary. Stir in cilantro. Transfer to a serving dish and garnish with cashew nuts. Serve hot.

Serves 4–6 (vegetarian menu) with rice and/or bread, 1 or more accompaniments, and Sweet-and-Sour Lentils (page 164)
Serves 4–6 (meat menu) with rice and/or bread, 1 or more accompaniments, and 1 chicken, meat or seafood main dish
Serves 6–8 (vegetarian menu) with rice and/or bread, 1 or more accompaniments, Sweet-and-Sour Lentils (page 164), and 1 other vegetarian main dish
Serves 6–8 (meat menu) with rice and/or bread, 1 or more accompaniments, 1 other vegetarian main dish, and 1 chicken, meat or seafood main dish

Rich tomatoes with cashew nuts (front),
coconut rice (back)

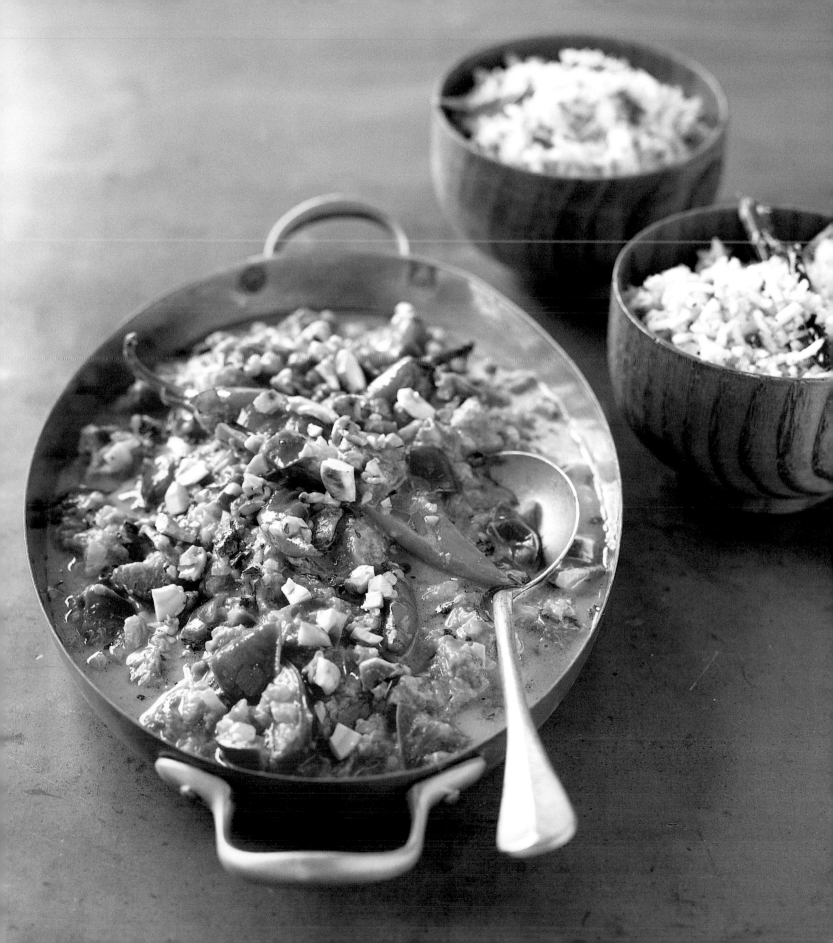

Sweet-and-sour lentils
Khatti dal

¹/₂ cup (3¹/₂ oz/100 g) split yellow lentils
2¹/₂ cups (20 fl oz/625 ml) water
1 teaspoon coriander seeds
1 teaspoon cumin seeds
2 tablespoons vegetable oil
1 yellow (brown) onion, halved and thinly sliced
1 teaspoon salt
1 teaspoon chili powder
1 teaspoon minced garlic
40 fresh curry leaves
2 ripe tomatoes, chopped
2 zucchini (courgettes), about 6 oz (180 g) total weight, chopped
1 cup (8 fl oz/250 ml) water
6¹/₂ oz (200 g) asparagus, tough ends removed and cut into ¹/₂ -inch (12-mm) pieces
1 teaspoon tamarind concentrate
1 teaspoon chickpea flour dissolved in ¹/₄ cup (2 fl oz/60 ml) water
Leaves from 1 bunch fresh cilantro (fresh coriander), chopped

Steamed Basmati Rice (page 141) and/or Home-style Bread (page 141) for serving
Onion Raita (page 168), Sesame Seed Chutney (page 168), Tomato Pickle (page 169) and/or Garlic and Red Chili Chutney (page 169) for serving

1. Rinse lentils. In a small saucepan, combine lentils and water, cover and bring to a boil over high heat. Reduce heat to medium, uncover and cook, stirring often, until lentils break down completely and all water is absorbed, 45–50 minutes. Mixture should be quite thick. Remove from heat and set aside.
2. In a spice grinder, combine coriander and cumin seeds and grind to a fine powder. In a saucepan, heat oil over medium–low heat. Add onion and salt and cook until onion is golden brown, 20–25 minutes. Add ground spices, chili powder, garlic and curry leaves and cook, stirring, for 2 minutes.
3. Add tomatoes, zucchini and water to pan, cover partially and cook over medium heat until vegetables are tender, about 15 minutes. Add asparagus and tamarind, stir well and cook, uncovered, until asparagus is tender, about 10 minutes longer.
4. Stir in cooked lentils and chickpea flour and cook over low heat, stirring, until mixture is well combined. Raise heat to high and allow mixture to come to a boil and thicken.
5. Taste and adjust seasoning with salt if necessary. Stir in cilantro and transfer to a serving dish, or garnish with cilantro. Serve hot.

Serves 4–6 (vegetarian menu) with rice and/or bread, 1 or more accompaniments, and 1 other vegetarian main dish
Serves 4–6 (meat) with rice and/or bread, 1 or more accompaniments, and 1 chicken, lamb or seafood main dish
Serves 6–8 (vegetarian menu) with rice and/or bread, 1 or more accompaniments, and 2 other vegetarian main dishes
Serves 6–8 (meat menu) with rice and/or bread, 1 or more accompaniments, 1 other vegetarian main dish, and 1 chicken, lamb or seafood main dish

Banana chilies in sesame sauce
Mirch ka salan

Vegetable oil for deep-frying,
plus 1/3 cup (3 fl oz/90 ml)
2 lb (1 kg) fresh banana chilies,
slit lengthwise and seeds removed
3 yellow (brown) onions, halved and
thinly sliced
1 teaspoon salt
1/4 cup (1 oz/30 g) Salan Masala
(page 31)
1 teaspoon grated fresh ginger
1 teaspoon minced garlic
40 fresh curry leaves
1/4 cup (2 fl oz/60 ml) water
3–4 teaspoons tamarind concentrate

Steamed Basmati Rice (page 141)
and/or Home-style Bread (page 141)
for serving
Onion Raita (page 168), Sesame Seed
Chutney (page 168), Tomato Pickle
(page 169), and/or Garlic and Red
Chili Chutney (page 169) for serving

Here, banana chilies are gently simmered in a salan, or spicy gravy.

1. Pour oil to a depth of 4 inches (10 cm) into a large, deep saucepan and heat to 350°F (180°C) on a deep-frying thermometer. Working in batches, add chilies and fry just until they change color, 30–60 seconds. Using a slotted spoon or tongs, transfer to a plate.
2. In a large saucepan, heat 1/3 cup (3 fl oz/90 ml) oil over medium–low heat. Add onions and salt and cook uncovered, stirring occasionally, until onions are dark golden brown, 20–25 minutes. Add masala, ginger and garlic and cook, stirring, for 2 minutes.
3. Add chilies, curry leaves and water to pan. Cook, uncovered, over medium–low heat until chilies are very soft, 10–15 minutes. Stir in tamarind to taste.
4. Taste and adjust seasoning with salt if necessary. Transfer to a serving dish and serve hot.

Serves 4–6 (vegetarian menu) with rice and/or bread, 1 or more accompaniments, and Sweet-and-Sour Lentils (page 164)
Serves 4–6 (meat menu) with rice and/or bread, 1 or more accompaniments, and 1 chicken, lamb or seafood main dish
Serves 6–8 (vegetarian menu) with rice and/or bread, 1 or more accompaniments, Sweet-and-Sour Lentils (page 164), and 1 other vegetarian main dish
Serves 6–8 (meat menu) with rice and/or bread, 1 or more accompaniments, 1 other vegetarian main dish, and 1 chicken, lamb or seafood main dish

Note: Banana chilies are about 6 inches (15 cm) long, mild to sweet, and green, yellow or red. Do not confuse them with the hotter Hungarian wax or yellow wax chili.

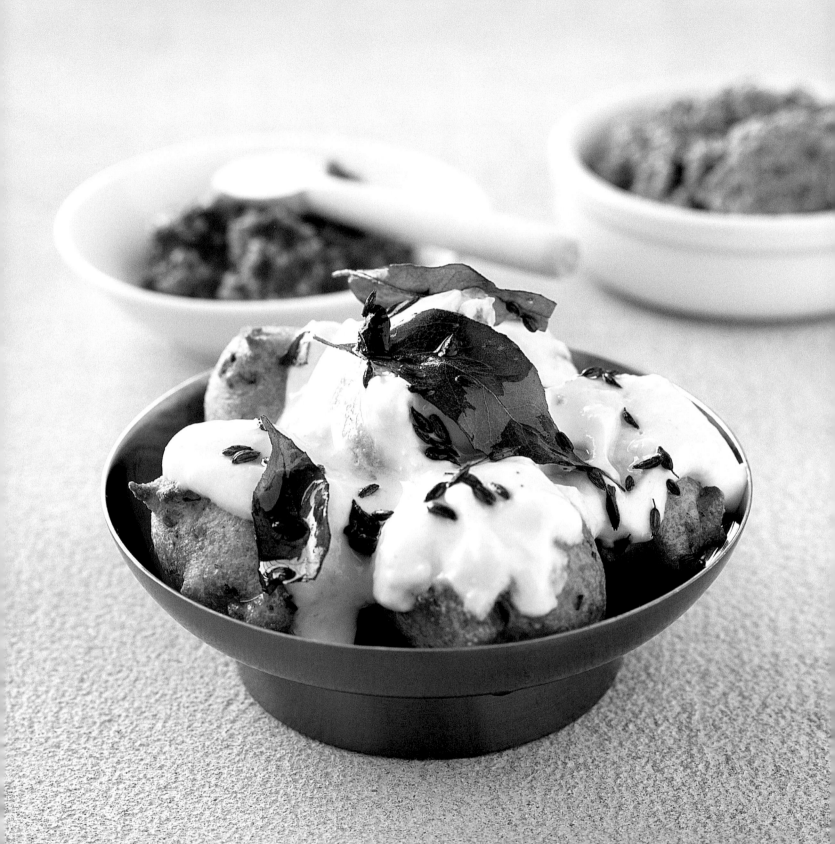

Chickpea dumplings in yogurt sauce
Dahi ki kadi

For Dumplings (Bhajiyas)
2/3 cup (3 oz/90 g) chickpea flour
2 fresh mild long green chilies, finely chopped
2 tablespoons chopped fresh cilantro (fresh coriander)
1/2 teaspoon baking soda
Pinch salt
4–5 tablespoons water
Vegetable oil for deep-frying

For Yogurt Sauce (Kadi)
2 cups (1 lb/500 g) plain whole-milk yogurt, whisked until smooth
2 tablespoons chickpea flour
1 1/2 teaspoons minced garlic
1 1/2 teaspoons grated fresh ginger
1/2 teaspoon ground turmeric
1 tablespoon desiccated coconut, dry-roasted on stove top and ground to fine powder in spice grinder
1 teaspoon salt

For Tempering (Bhagar)
2 tablespoons vegetable oil
1 teaspoon cumin seeds
2 dried red chilies, broken into small pieces
20 fresh curry leaves

Steamed Basmati Rice (page 141) and/or Home-style Bread (page 141), Onion Raita (page 168), Sesame Seed Chutney (page 168), Tomato Pickle (page 169), and/or Garlic and Red Chili Chutney (page 169)

1. To make bhajiyas: In a bowl, combine chickpea flour, chilies, cilantro, baking soda and salt. Stir in enough water to make a thick batter. Pour oil to a depth of 4 inches (10 cm) into a large, deep saucepan and heat to 350°F (180°C) on a deep-frying thermometer. Working in batches, carefully drop teaspoonfuls of mixture into hot oil and cook until golden brown, 3–4 minutes. Using a slotted spoon, transfer to paper towels to drain.
2. To make kadi: In a bowl, stir together yogurt and chickpea flour until smooth and well combined. Stir in garlic, ginger and turmeric until well mixed and then mix in coconut and salt until evenly distributed. Place over low heat and stir until mixture comes to a simmer.
3. To make bhagar: In a small frying pan, heat oil over medium heat. Add cumin seeds and cook until they start to pop, 1–2 minutes. Stir in chilies and curry leaves and cook until leaves crisp slightly, 1–2 minutes. Remove from heat.
4. Transfer bhajiyas to a serving dish and pour over kadi. Top with bhagar and serve immediately.

Serves 4–6 (vegetarian menu) with rice and/or bread, 1 or more accompaniments, and Sweet-and-Sour Lentils (page 164)
Serves 4–6 (meat menu) with rice and/or bread, 1 or more accompaniments, and 1 chicken, meat or seafood main dish
Serves 6–8 (vegetarian menu) with rice and/or bread, 1 or more accompaniments, Sweet-and-Sour Lentils (page 164), and 1 other vegetarian main dish
Serves 6–8 (meat menu) with rice and/or bread, 1 or more accompaniments, 1 other vegetarian main dish, and 1 chicken, meat or seafood main dish

Chickpea dumplings (front),
garlic and red chili chutney (back left),
sesame seed chutney (back right)

Accompaniments

Onion raita
Pyaaz-ka-raita

2 yellow (brown) onions, halved and thinly sliced
1 fresh mild long green chili, finely chopped
1/2 teaspoon cumin seeds, ground in spice grinder
Juice of 1/2 lemon
1 tablespoon chopped fresh cilantro (fresh coriander)
1 cup (8 oz/250 g) plain whole-milk yogurt, whisked until smooth
Salt

1. In a bowl, combine onions, chili, cumin, lemon juice, cilantro and yogurt and stir well to combine. Season to taste with salt.
2. Serve soon after making.

Serves 6–8

Sesame seed chutney
Til-ki-chatni

1/4 cup (1 oz/30 g) sesame seeds
3 tablespoons unsalted raw peanuts
6 fresh mild long green chilies, roughly chopped
2 yellow (brown) onions, chopped
1 tablespoon minced garlic
1/2 cup (1/2 oz/15 g) fresh cilantro (fresh coriander) leaves
2 teaspoons tamarind concentrate
Salt

1. Preheat oven to 350°F (180°C/Gas 4). Spread sesame seeds on a small rimmed baking sheet. Place in oven and toast until golden, 5–6 minutes. Transfer to a small food processor. Leave oven on.
2. Spread peanuts on same baking sheet, place in oven and toast until golden, 8–10 minutes. Add to food processor and let cool slightly.
3. Process sesame seeds and peanuts until finely ground. Add chilies, onions, garlic, cilantro and tamarind and process until well combined. Season to taste with salt.
4. Transfer to a serving dish and serve. Store leftover chutney in an airtight container in refrigerator for up to 2 weeks.

Makes 1 cup (8 fl oz/250 ml)

Tomato pickle
Tamartar achar

1 tablespoon dry mustard
(mustard powder)
1 teaspoon fenugreek seeds,
ground in spice grinder
1/4 teaspoon powdered asafetida
1 1/2 teaspoons chili powder
5 tablespoons vegetable oil
1 1/2 lb (750 g) firm, ripe tomatoes,
quartered
1 teaspoon tamarind concentrate
1 teaspoon ground turmeric

For Tempering
3 tablespoons vegetable oil
2 dried red chilies
1 tablespoon roasted split chickpeas
1 tablespoon split white lentils
(optional)
1 tablespoon black or brown
mustard seeds
2 teaspoons salt

1. In a small, nonstick frying pan, dry-roast dry mustard, fenugreek, asafetida and chili powder over medium heat until fragrant, 2–3 minutes. Remove pan from heat.
2. In a heavy-bottomed saucepan, heat oil over low heat. Add tomatoes and cook until they break down, 30–40 minutes. Remove pan from heat and let cool slightly.
3. In a food processor, combine tomatoes, roasted spices, tamarind and turmeric and process until well combined.
4. To make tempering: Rinse and dry saucepan, place over medium heat and add oil. When hot, add chilies, roasted split chickpeas, lentils if using and mustard seeds and cook, stirring, until seeds start to pop and chickpeas and lentils turn dark brown, 2–3 minutes. Stir in salt and remove from heat.
5. Add tomato mixture to pan and stir until well combined. Return to medium heat and simmer, uncovered, until mixture thickens, about 15 minutes. (The thickness of the mixture will depend on the juiciness and ripeness of tomatoes you use; you may not need to reduce the sauce again if it is a good consistency.)
6. Serve at room temperature. Store leftover pickle in an airtight container in refrigerator for up to 2 weeks.

Makes about 2 cups

Garlic and red chili chutney
Lahsan lal mirch ki chatni

20 dried red chilies
Boiling water as needed
3 tablespoons minced garlic
2 teaspoons grated jaggery or
dark brown sugar
Juice of 1 lime
Salt

1. Place chilies in a large heatproof bowl and add boiling water to cover. Set aside until chilies soften, about 1 hour.
2. Drain chilies and place in a small food processor. Process until finely chopped. Add garlic, jaggery or brown sugar and lime juice and process until well combined.
3. Transfer to a small bowl and season to taste with salt. Serve immediately. Store leftover chutney in an airtight container in refrigerator for up to 2 weeks.

Makes about 1/4 cup

Desserts

Bread and butter pudding
Shahi tukra

6 slices white bread
²/₃ cup (5 oz/150 g) unsalted butter
3 cups (24 fl oz/750 ml) evaporated milk
¹/₄ cup (2 oz/60 g) sugar
¹/₄ teaspoon saffron threads, soaked in 2 tablespoons warm whole milk for 10 minutes
¹/₂ teaspoon ground green cardamom pods (ground in spice grinder)
1 tablespoon unsalted pistachio nuts, finely chopped

This is the Central Indian version of the Hyderabadi classic bread and butter pudding *(double ka meetha)*.

1. Cut crusts off bread slices, and cut each slice into 2 triangles. In a large frying pan, heat butter over medium heat. When butter starts to foam, add a few triangles of bread and cook, turning once, until golden brown, 3–4 minutes on each side. Remove from pan and repeat with remaining bread triangles.
2. In a heavy-bottomed saucepan, combine milk and sugar. Place over low heat and heat, stirring, until sugar dissolves and milk is hot. Remove pan from heat and stir in saffron and milk and cardamom.
3. Place 3 triangles of bread in each individual bowl. Pour milk mixture over bread triangles, dividing evenly. Refrigerate for 15 minutes to allow bread to soak up some of milk mixture and to chill.
4. Sprinkle bread with pistachio nuts and serve.

Serves 4

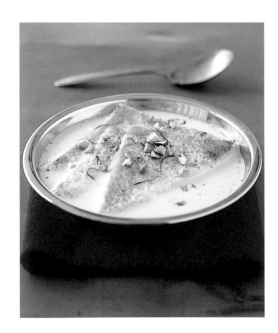

Whole-wheat halwa

Aate-ka-halwa

1/3 cup (3 fl oz/90 ml) vegetable oil
1/3 cup (3 oz/90 g) unsalted butter
2 whole cloves
3 green cardamom pods
1 cup (5 oz/150 g) whole-wheat (wholemeal) flour
3/4 cup (6 oz/180 g) sugar
3 cups (24 fl oz/750 ml) boiling water
Pinch saffron threads, soaked in
2 tablespoons warm whole milk for 10 minutes
2 tablespoons raisins, chopped
2 tablespoons chopped unsalted roasted cashew nuts or blanched almonds

1. In a heavy-bottomed saucepan, heat oil and butter over medium heat. When butter has melted, add cloves and cardamom and cook, stirring, until fragrant, 2–3 minutes. Stir in flour, reduce heat to low and cook, stirring, until mixture is a nutty brown, about 15 minutes.
2. In a heatproof bowl, combine sugar and boiling water and stir until sugar dissolves. Gradually add sugar mixture to flour mixture while stirring constantly and then cook, stirring, until mixture starts to stick to pan, 4–5 minutes.
3. Remove pan from heat and stir in saffron and milk. Serve hot, or reheat gently just before serving. Top with raisins and nuts just before serving.

Serves 6–8

Index

Guide to weights and measures

The metric weights and metric fluid measures used in this book are those of Standards Australia. All cup and spoon measurements are level:
- The Australian Standard measuring cup has a capacity of 250 millilitres (250 ml).
- The Australian Standard tablespoon has a capacity of 20 millilitres (20 ml).

In all recipes metric equivalents of imperial measures are shown in parentheses e.g. 1 lb (500 g) beef. For successful cooking use either metric or imperial weights and measures—do not mix the two.

Weights

Imperial	Metric
$^1/_3$ oz	10 g
$^1/_2$ oz	15 g
$^3/_4$ oz	20 g
1 oz	30 g
2 oz	60 g
3 oz	90 g
4 oz ($^1/_4$ lb)	125 g
5 oz ($^1/_3$ lb)	150 g
6 oz	180 g
7 oz	220 g
8 oz ($^1/_2$ lb)	250 g
9 oz	280 g
10 oz	300 g
11 oz	330 g
12 oz ($^3/_4$ lb)	375 g
16 oz (1 lb)	500 g
2 lb	1 kg
3 lb	1.5 kg
4 lb	2 kg

Volume

Imperial	Metric	Cup
1 fl oz	30 ml	
2 fl oz	60 ml	$^1/_4$
3 fl oz	90 ml	$^1/_3$
4 fl oz	125 ml	$^1/_2$
5 fl oz	150 ml	$^2/_3$
6 fl oz	180 ml	$^3/_4$
8 fl oz	250 ml	1
10 fl oz	300 ml	$1^1/_4$
12 fl oz	375 ml	$1^1/_2$
13 fl oz	400 ml	$1^2/_3$
14 fl oz	440 ml	$1^3/_4$
16 fl oz	500 ml	2
24 fl oz	750 ml	3
32 fl oz	1 L	4

Oven temperature guide

The Celsius (°C) and Fahrenheit (°F) temperatures in this chart apply to most electric ovens. Decrease by 25°F or 10°C for a gas oven or refer to the manufacturer's temperature guide. For temperatures below 325°F (160°C), do not decrease the given temperature.

Oven description	°C	°F	Gas Mark
Cool	110	225	$^1/_4$
	130	250	$^1/_2$
Very slow	140	275	1
	150	300	2
Slow	170	325	3
Moderate	180	350	4
	190	375	5
Moderately Hot	200	400	6
Fairly Hot	220	425	7
Hot	230	450	8
Very Hot	240	475	9
Extremely Hot	250	500	10

Useful conversions

$^1/_4$ teaspoon	1.25 ml
$^1/_2$ teaspoon	2.5 ml
1 teaspoon	5 ml
1 Australian tablespoon	20 ml (4 teaspoons)
1 UK/US tablespoon	15 ml (3 teaspoons)

Butter/Shortening		
1 tablespoon	$^1/_2$ oz	15 g
$1^1/_2$ tablespoons	$^3/_4$ oz	20 g
2 tablespoons	1 oz	30 g
3 tablespoons	$1^1/_2$ oz	45 g

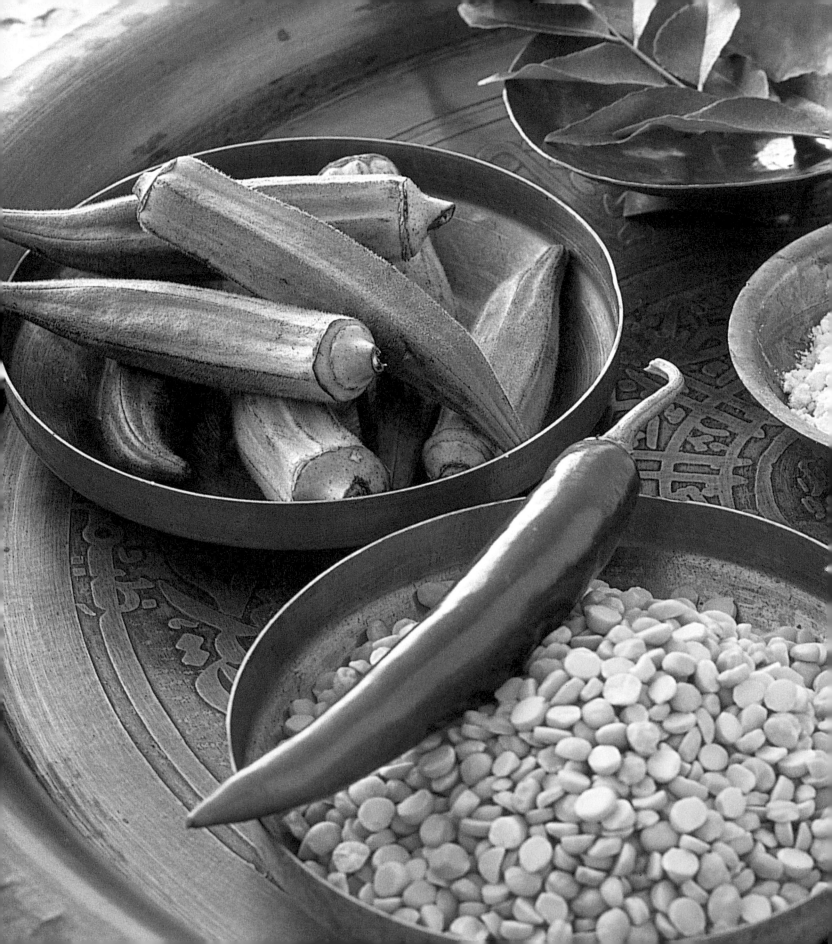